Clinical Handbook of
Chinese Medicine

Clinical Handbook of
Chinese Medicine

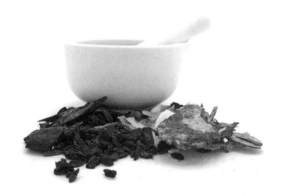

Bob Xu
American Chinese Medicine Association, USA

Chun-Su Yuan
University of Chicago, USA

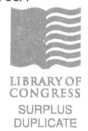

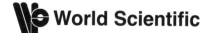 **World Scientific**

NEW JERSEY · LONDON · SINGAPORE · BEIJING · SHANGHAI · HONG KONG · TAIPEI · CHENNAI

Published by

World Scientific Publishing Co. Pte. Ltd.

5 Toh Tuck Link, Singapore 596224

USA office: 27 Warren Street, Suite 401-402, Hackensack, NJ 07601

UK office: 57 Shelton Street, Covent Garden, London WC2H 9HE

Library of Congress Cataloging-in-Publication Data
Xu, Bob.
    Clinical handbook of Chinese medicine / by Bob Xu, Chun-Su Yuan.
       p. ; cm.
    Includes bibliographical references and index.
    ISBN 978-9814366120 (hardcover : alk. paper)
    I. Yuan, Chun-Su. II. Title.
    [DNLM: 1. Medicine, Chinese Traditional--Handbooks. WB 39]

    610.951--dc23
                                      2012046515

British Library Cataloguing-in-Publication Data
A catalogue record for this book is available from the British Library.

Typeset by Stallion Press
Email: enquiries@stallionpress.com

Printed in Singapore by World Scientific Printers.

Note to Readers and How to Use this Book

Chinese medicine (CM) is an individualized medicine, very different from Western medicine (WM). CM herbs should be prescribed with the principle of *bian zheng lun zhi*, treating each patient individually, based on the patient's specific diagnosed conditions. Thus, CM herbs cannot be used in the same way as WM drugs.

For this reason, all formulations in this book are strictly general examples. They should not be administered to patients without being prescribed from qualified CM doctors. It is erroneous to massively manufacture CM herbs as dietary supplements or medications. Allowing patients to take CM herbs in this manner may cause serious, adverse events. Numerous reports show instances of CM utilized incorrectly. For example, in the 1990s, many people suffered from kidney failure and other adverse events after taking Chinese herbs for weight loss. Approximately 10 years ago, a number of people died and thousands suffered side effects from using a CM herb, ephedra, as a dietary supplement. These incidents were caused by the intake of herbs without the prescription of CM qualified doctors or the incorrect use of CM. These events can be avoided if qualified CM doctors prescribe CM herbs based on the *bain zheng lun zhi* principle.

Due to historical reasons as well as language and cultural differences, many terms in CM do not have exact counterparts in English. Direct translation of these CM terms into English may distort or lose their original meanings. This English language expression poses a challenge to the authors. In order to obtain a correct interpretation and a good understanding of the text, the reader should be aware that there is a disjoint between CM terms and English terminology. To resolve this issue, three appendices have been provided at the end of this handbook.

Appendix I. Acupuncture Points — Since acupuncture points do not have counterparts in English, we used pinyin forms, the official phonetic system for transcribing the sound of Chinese characters into Latin script. The meanings of pinyin forms are explained.

Appendix II. Glossary — For all CM terms other than acupuncture points and herbal formulations, pinyin forms are used and explained.

Appendix III. Index of Formulae — For herbal formulations that do not have exact counterparts in English, pinyin forms are used and explained.

Thus, whenever you meet a term that is unfamiliar in English, using appendices will be helpful. Frequent reference to these appendices is valuable to understand the meaning of CM terminologies.

Table of Contents

PART I

OVERVIEW

1. Introduction

Chinese medicine (CM), also called traditional Chinese medicine (TCM), is an integral part of Chinese culture and history. It originated from, grows, develops, and evolves side by side with Chinese culture and history, and in return, Chinese medicine has enriched Chinese culture and history. Due to this close relationship, it is necessary to understand Chinese culture and history in order to understand Chinese medicine.

2. Chinese History vs. Chinese Medicine

Generally speaking, Chinese medicine is composed of two parts: theory and practice. The practice of Chinese medicine is the basis and foundation of its theory. The theory of Chinese medicine is a summary and sublimation of the practice.

Medically, the theory and practice of Chinese medicine are closely related. However, during the course of the history of Chinese medicine, the two parts did not evolve side by side. The practice of Chinese medicine started much earlier than the formation of Chinese medical theory.

The origin of Chinese medical practice was closely associated with the activities of Chinese ancestors in the primitive era. During that era, the basic survival needs of human beings were not guaranteed.

Diseases, illnesses, wounds, etc., were constantly threatening the survival of Chinese ancestors. They faced these threats everyday. Basic survival was a huge challenge. In that hostile environment, they tried every possible means available to survive the diseases, illnesses, wounds, etc.

Because one of the most pressing tasks at that time was to fight the diseases, illnesses, wounds, etc., the need for a primitive medicine became evident. In other words, whenever there was a human being, there was a need for medicine. The need for medicine was a top priority for Chinese ancestors of that era.[1]

As a result, the practice of Chinese medicine started at the very beginning of Chinese history. In fact, the practice of Chinese medicine began as soon as Chinese history began.

The earliest practice of Chinese medicine, however, was not as sophisticated and advanced as the practice of Chinese medicine today. The early practice of Chinese medicine was primarily composed of simple, random, and non-purposeful behaviors. Many of them could be described as subconscious, unintentional, trial-and-error, and non-systematic approaches.

Since there was no printed or electronic documentation at that time, there was no means of keeping a record of practices in that era. Therefore, the exact date of the start of Chinese medical practice was not documented. However, since the practice of Chinese medicine began as soon as Chinese history started, it is possible to derive the history of Chinese medicine from our knowledge of Chinese history. So far, most of the knowledge on Chinese medicine has been obtained through historical study and research on Chinese culture and history.

3. Misunderstandings of Chinese Medical History

Due to cultural and language differences, there exist some misunderstandings of the history of Chinese medicine in the early English-language accounts of Chinese medicine. Many misunderstandings originated from the book *Huang Di Nei Jing*.

Huang Di Nei Jing is the earliest book available to date which deals with established Chinese medical theory. This book was the product of many authors spanning several generations. The names of the authors are unknown and the exact times when it was started and finished are unclear. It

---

[1]In Chinese history, there was no such term as *Chinese medicine*. Because there was only one medicine in China at that time, only *medicine* was used. The term *medicine* referred to Chinese medicine.

is generally believed that the book was written from the Spring and Autumn Period (770–476 B.C.) to the Warring States Period (475–221 B.C.).

Many English-language accounts of Chinese medicine regarded this book as the beginning of Chinese medicine. However, this is a misunderstanding of Chinese medical history.

Huang Di Nei Jing is a comprehensive encyclopedia-type reference book containing established Chinese medical theory. However, Chinese medicine could not have started with such a comprehensive reference book. Chinese medicine must have started with some primitive publications, documents, and other books first. After the primitive publications, documents, and books had accumulated to a certain degree, and when the knowledge of Chinese medicine had accumulated to a certain level, only then could this encyclopedia of the established theory of Chinese medicine be possible.

Therefore, before *Huang Di Nei Jing,* there must have been many other primitive and specialized publications, documents, and books on Chinese medicine. Although they were not preserved, they played very important transitional roles in the formation of Chinese medical theory. *Huang Di Nei Jing* is only a summary of the knowledge established before that era.

4. Obstacles in Chinese Medical History

Living in the contemporary era, we take for granted the many conveniences we enjoy. Since we have no experience of life in the primitive era, it is difficult for us to imagine what it was like then.

The following are the obstacles and difficulties faced in the history of Chinese medicine, which either slowed down or restricted the growth and development of Chinese medicine from primitive practices to the established theory.

(1) *Language*

In the primitive era, there was no well-established standard language in China. People in different parts of China spoke very different dialects and even those in the same province could not understand each other. They could not speak, communicate, or exchange ideas with each other as effectively as we do today.

As a result, the knowledge of Chinese medicine developed in one part of China would be restricted to that area for a very long time before being exchanged with people in other places. This severely slowed and limited the growth and development of Chinese medicine.

(2) *Documentation*

In the primitive era, there was no pen, paper, printing, publishing, or electronic recording techniques. Therefore, knowledge of Chinese medicine could not be documented and shared. The knowledge of Chinese medicine in that era could only be passed on orally. This also severely limited the growth and development of Chinese medicine.

(3) *Publication*

Even after oracle-bone script (jia gu wen), pen, and paper were developed, there was still no means of publication, so all books were single-copy. Knowledge of Chinese medicine could not be disseminated as effectively as today. This also severely limited the growth and development of Chinese medicine.

(4) *Preservation*

One important issue relating to single-copy books at that time was that if a book was lost, all of the information in that book would be permanently lost. This happened many times in the history of Chinese medicine. A single-copy book could be lost either through accidents, disasters, or through natural decaying processes.

Because paper older than 2,000 years decays completely, most books and documents from over 2,000 years ago are no longer available. As a result, most Chinese medical books and documents before *Huang Di Nei Jing* are not preserved.

Once a single-copy book is lost, all of the information in that book is lost permanently. It might take many generations to re-discover that lost knowledge. In some cases, the knowledge in the book might be lost forever. One example is the lost books of Hua Tuo. Up to today, the information lost in Hua Tuo's books still has not been recovered, developed, or re-invented. This is not only a heavy loss for Chinese medicine, but also a heavy loss for humanity.

Hua Tuo's books are only one known case. In most other cases, we do not know how much Chinese medicine has suffered and how much knowledge has been lost throughout history due to the loss of single-copy books.

Each loss of a book would slow down the growth and development of Chinese medicine. Therefore, the issue of single-copy books is another factor that severely delayed the development and growth of Chinese medicine.

(5) *Transportation*

In the primitive era, there were no cars, trains, ships, airplanes, etc. Therefore, the exchange between people was very restricted. As a result, in many parts of China, people did not interact with other areas and could not understand each other for a long time. Thus, the knowledge of Chinese medicine developed in one area could not be shared with people in other areas effectively. This was another factor that severely restricted and limited the growth and development of Chinese medicine.

(6) *Communication*

In the primitive era, there was no mail service, no post office, no electricity, no radio, no television, no phone, no computer, no Internet, etc. It was very difficult and inefficient for people to exchange knowledge of Chinese medicine with each other.

The poor communication conditions were another factor that severely slowed down the development and growth of Chinese medicine.

Considering all the obstacles to the growth and development of Chinese medicine, it is reasonable to believe that a very long time was needed for the evolution of Chinese medicine from its practice in the beginning to the formation of the current theory. In other words, the beginning of Chinese medical practice was much earlier than the beginning of Chinese medical theory.

5. Milestones in Chinese Medical History

There were many important events in the history of Chinese medicine. The following are some historical milestones.

(1) *Beginning of Chinese Medical Practice*

According to historical studies and research, the currently available and documented period of the consanguine family in China included the following: Yuan Mou Ren (Yunnan Province) which existed about 1,700,000 years ago; Lan Tian Ren (Shaanxi Province) which existed about 800,000 years ago; Beijing Ren (Beijing) which existed about 690,000 years ago; and He Xian Ren (Anhui Province) which existed about 690,000 years ago.

During this period, Chinese ancestors ate everything available to them in that environment. They gathered primitive experience and knowledge on all the foods they ate through trial and error. They found some plants, leaves, fruits, seeds, roots, etc., that could cause diarrhea, vomiting, coma, aggravation of their existing conditions, or even death, while other plants, leaves, fruits, seeds, roots, etc., could relieve their symptoms, treat their diseases and illnesses, or heal their wounds. These experiences and knowledge were then directly applied to combat diseases, illnesses, and wounds. This was the origin and primitive practice of Chinese herbal medicine.

Fire and stone tools were discovered and developed during this period. People gradually found that fire could make them feel comfortable at night and in cold weather. It also could relieve some symptoms. Thus, fire was applied purposefully to relieve some conditions and symptoms, and to treat some diseases and illnesses. This was the origin and primitive practice of moxibustion.

In the course of work and daily activities, people found that unintentional falls and sitting on the ground or stones alleviated some pre-existing pain or other symptoms. Gradually, people started to use stones purposefully to press or hit certain positions on the body in order to relieve pain and other symptoms. To make this procedure more effective, the bian shi (the earliest stone needle) was developed and used in a purposeful manner to relieve some symptoms and pains. This was the origin and primitive practice of acupuncture.

(2) *Invention of Bone Needle, Tooth Needle, and Advanced Stone Needle*

The matrilineal society in China started about 200,000 years ago. It included Da Li Ren (Shaanxi Province), Ma Ba Ren (Guangdong Province), Chang Yang Ren (Hubei Province), and Ding Cun Ren (Shanxi Province).

During this time, stone tools became more delicate. The bian shi was improved. The bone needle, tooth needle, etc., were developed during this period.

(3) *Advanced Practices of Chinese Medicine*

China's matrilineal society entered into its prosperous period around 8,000 years ago. Many clusters of cultures were developed around this time. It included the Pei Li Gang Culture, He Mu Du Culture, Yang Shao Culture, Qing Lian Gang Culture, and Ma Jia Bang Culture.

During this period, the bian shi and bone needle became more advanced. Purposeful agriculture of herbs and plants and animal husbandry were developed. Pottery was invented during this period. Decoction became available. These advancements facilitated more effective practices of Chinese medicine on a larger scale.

(4) *Invention of Metal Needle*

China's patrilineal society started around 5,000 years ago. It included the Long Shan Culture, Da Wen Kou Culture, Liang Zhu Culture, and Qi Jia Culture.

During this time, metallurgy was developed. Metal needles became available during this period. This improved the acupuncture technique, bringing it to a more advanced level.

(5) *Earliest Available Written Documentation of the Practice of Chinese Medicine*

The earliest available written documentation of the practice of Chinese medicine was found in some legends documented in ancient Chinese books. Examples of those legends include the legend of "Fu Yi Making Nine Needles", the legend of "Fu Yi Trying Hundreds of Herbs", the legend of "Shen Nong Trying Hundreds of Herbs", and the legend of "Huang Di Teaching Medicine."

These legends document the practice of Chinese medicine in that era. The figures in these legends were either heads of ancient Chinese tribes or famous Chinese leaders. Because the heads of ancient tribes or leaders were unlikely to be doctors or practitioners of Chinese medicine, these legends probably just borrowed those well-known people's names to document, represent, and reflect the status and achievement of Chinese medicine practiced by many doctors and practitioners of Chinese medicine during that period.

Because these legends existed long before the earliest books that could be preserved to today, the exact times when these legends started and existed are unknown. It is generally believed that these legends existed around the matrilineal society to the patrilineal society.

(6) *Earliest Available Written Documentation of Chinese Herbal Medicine*

The earliest available written documentation of Chinese herbal medicine is *Shang Shu*. The author and time of the book are unknown. It was probably written by many authors and spanned a long period of time during the Zhou Dynasty (1066–476 B.C.). Books before that era could not be preserved and are all unavailable now.

(7) *Earliest Available Written Documentation of Acupuncture*

The earliest available written documentation of acupuncture consists of two books, *Zu Bi Shi Yi Mai Jiu Jing* and *Yin Yang Shi Yi Mai Jiu Jing*. These two books were discovered in Ma Wang Dui (Changsha, Hunan Province).

The authors and detailed dates of when the books were written are unknown. However, it is known that these two books were written earlier than *Huang Di Nei Jing*.

(8) *Earliest Available Written Documentation of Obstetrics and Gynecology in Chinese Medicine*

The earliest written documentation available today of obstetrics and gynecology in Chinese medicine was written in jia gu wen around the Shang Dynasty (1400 B.C.) and was discovered in Yin Xu (Anyang, Henan Province).

(9) *Earliest Available Written Documentation of Pediatrics in Chinese Medicine*

The earliest written documentation available today of a doctor of Chinese medicine specializing in pediatrics is of Bian Que, also known as Qin Yue Ren, Lu Yi, who lived around 400 B.C. He was one of the greatest doctors in the history of Chinese medicine. There may have been other Chinese medical pediatric doctors before him, but since books before that era could not be preserved, Bian Que is regarded as the earliest Chinese medical pediatric doctor known today.

(10) *Earliest Available Written Documentation of Surgery in Chinese Medicine*

The earliest written documentation available today of surgery in Chinese medicine was written in jia gu wen around the Shang Dynasty (1400 B.C.) and was discovered in Yin Xu (Anyang, Henan Province).

(11) *Earliest Available Book on Chinese Medicine*

The earliest book available today dealing with many fields of Chinese medicine is *Wu Shi Er Bing Fang*. This book was discovered in Ma Wang Dui (Changsha, Hunan Province).

The author and exact date of when the book was written are not known yet. But it is known that this book was written earlier than *Huang Di Nei Jing*.

(12) *Earliest Available Comprehensive Encyclopedia*
     of Chinese Medicine

From the Spring and Autumn Period (770–476 B.C.) to the Warring States Period (475–221 B.C.), based on the advancement of Chinese medicine and many books written before that era, multiple authors wrote *Huang Di Nei Jing* over a period of several generations. This book borrowed Huang Di's name (one of China's leaders in that era). However, the book was not Huang Di's work. The actual names of the authors are unknown.

This book contains two parts: *Su Wen* and *Ling Shu*. It is the earliest comprehensive encyclopedia-type reference book on Chinese medicine available today. It includes many achievements of Chinese medicine that had accumulated by that time. It contains established principles, theories, and methodologies of Chinese medicine.

Many English-language accounts of Chinese medicine regard this book as the beginning of Chinese medicine. This is a misunderstanding, since both the practice and the theory of Chinese medicine started much earlier. This book was only an intermediate summary of the achievements in Chinese medicine that had accumulated by that era. Chinese medicine did not arise in one step with such a comprehensive reference book.

(13) *Earliest Available Book on Chinese Herbal Medicine*

Between the Spring and Autumn Period (770–476 B.C.) and the Warring States Period (475–221 B.C.), another important book on Chinese herbal medicine, *Shen Nong Ben Cao Jing*, was written. This book was based on the legend of "Shen Nong Trying Hundreds of Herbs." The book was also written by many authors, spanning several generations. The actual names of those authors are unknown. The authors just borrowed Shen Nong's name in memory of the famous hero in the legend.

This book is the earliest one on Chinese herbal medicine available today. The original copy of this book was lost in the Tang Dynasty. The current copy was extracted from *Zheng Lei Ben Cao* and *Ben Cao Gang Mu*.

(14) *Earliest Available Book on Treatment*
    Based on CM Diagnosis

Around the Eastern Han Dynasty, Zhang Zhong Jing wrote *Shang Han Za Bing Lun*, which established the principle of treatment based on CM Diagnosis. This book was divided into two parts, *Shang Han Lun* and *Jin Gui Yao Lue*, in the Jin Dynasty.

(15) *Earliest Available Written Documentation*
    of Ophthalmology in Chinese Medicine

The earliest written documentation available today of ophthalmology in Chinese medicine was written in jia gu wen around the Shang Dynasty (1400 B.C.) and was discovered in Yin Xu (Anyang, Henan Province).

(16) *Earliest Available Written Documentation*
    of Otorhinolaryngology in Chinese Medicine

The earliest written documentation available today of otorhinolaryngology in Chinese medicine was written in jia gu wen around the Shang Dynasty (1400 B.C.) and was discovered in Yin Xu (Anyang, Henan Province).

(17) *Earliest Available Written Documentation*
    of Traumatology in Chinese Medicine

The earliest written documentation available today of traumatology in Chinese medicine was written in jia gu wen around the Shang Dynasty (1400 B.C.) and was discovered in Yin Xu (Anyang, Henan Province).

(18) *World's First Book on Pathology*

In the Sui Dynasty (A.D. 610), Chao Yuan Fang and other authors wrote *Zhu Bing Yuan Hou Lun*. This book was the world's first book on pathology in medicine.

(19) *World's Earliest Medical School*

The world's first public medical school was called Tai Yi Shu. Tai Yi Shu was established in the Sui Dynasty (A.D. 581–618) by China's Sui government. It was the earliest government-run institution for Chinese medical doctor (CMD) teaching, education, and training. It was established more than 1,000 years before Harvard Medical School.

Before Tai Yi Shu, many private CMD medical schools existed. Since those private medical schools were not very well documented, it is difficult to trace their origins. Therefore, the well-documented Tai Yi Shu is recognized and regarded as the world's first medical school. However, strictly speaking, Tai Yi Shu was only the first government-run medical school. The actual first medical school would have been the earliest private medical school, which existed before Tai Yi Shu.

(20) *World's First Medical Degree*

The Chinese medical doctor (CMD) degree issued by Tai Yi Shu is regarded as the world's first medical degree.

(21) *World's First Government Pharmacopeia*

In the Tang Dynasty (A.D. 659), the Chinese government published *Xin Xiu Ben Cao*. This was the first government-issued pharmacopeia in the world.

These are some of the milestones in the history of Chinese medicine. There were many other important events, books, and doctors in the history of Chinese medicine, but because they could not be documented and preserved, they were permanently lost. Due to this reason, only the milestones known to us today are listed. The actual milestones of the history of Chinese medicine will remain myths forever.

6. Pre-scientific, Qualitative, and Philosophical Medicine

Chinese medicine was developed long before the advent of contemporary science. Therefore, it can be regarded as a *pre-scientific medicine*. Here, the term *pre-scientific* is relative to the current definition of *science*.

Because Chinese medicine was developed long before the advent of mathematics, it can be regarded as a *qualitative medicine*. At the time when Chinese medicine was formulated, there were no mathematical tools available. As a result, Chinese medicine was mainly built on qualitative variables and parameters. This, however, does not mean that Chinese medicine excludes mathematics. On the contrary, Chinese medicine calls for new mathematics. *Mathematical herbal medicine* has elucidated the relationship between Chinese medicine and mathematics.

Because Chinese medicine was founded on ancient Chinese philosophies, it can be regarded as a *philosophical medicine*. The fact that Chinese medicine was built on Chinese philosophies also reflects that Chinese medicine is an integral part of Chinese culture and history.

The fundamental philosophy of Chinese medicine is *yi jing* (also translated as *I Ching* in English). The application philosophies of Chinese medicine are the *yin yang theory, five elements theory*, etc.

7. Complexity of Chinese Medicine

Chinese medicine is a very complex medical system. The complexity can be elucidated from the following aspects.

(1) *Theoretical Complexity*

In allopathic medicine, a pharmaceutical drug usually contains one or a few active ingredients. Models studying pharmaceutical drugs belong to a linear system or a single-body, nonlinear system. Differential equations for the pharmacokinetics of these systems are solvable. Therefore, it is possible to control and analyze the chemical drug's process analytically and accurately in Western medicine's pharmaceutical research.

However, the situation in Chinese medicine is very different. A single Chinese herb usually contains dozens or hundreds of ingredients. A formula usually contains hundreds or even thousands of ingredients. During decoction (a process of boiling the herbs together in a liquid such as water), there are cross-reactions between these ingredients which make the decoction even more complicated. *In vivo*, the pharmacokinetics of herbal medicine usually involves many ingredients. Some of them may act together and couple with each other. As a result, models for the underlying process of Chinese medicine fall into multi-body, nonlinear systems.

Currently, the partial differential equations for the multi-body, nonlinear system of Chinese medicine cannot be solved accurately. Therefore, there is no mathematical tool to study the pharmacokinetic processes of Chinese medicine *in vivo* analytically and accurately. As a result, the system of Chinese medicine appears to be a black box.

This is the theoretical difficulty underlying the modern scientific study of Chinese medicine.

(2) *Experimental Complexity*

In order to maintain the multi-body, nonlinear nature of Chinese medicine, experimental study of Chinese medicine should be carried out in the intact formula environment.

The experimental difficulty in conducting a systematic and rigorous study of Chinese medicine is the control of variable settings. Because conclusions from studying an isolated ingredient may be different from those from studying a formula, it is inappropriate to draw conclusions based on studies of isolated ingredients.

Thus, it may be inappropriate to conclude which ingredient is active and which is not, simply based on the study of isolated ingredients. A complete, rigorous study of a formula demands a full study of all variable settings in the formula state.

Because the ingredient variable is more accurate than the herb variable, the study should concentrate on the variables of ingredients. However, this is sometimes very difficult to implement. For example, if a formula consists of 50 ingredients (this is a conservative estimate) and each variable (ingredient) takes on 10 different values (e.g. 10 different "strengths") during the control study, there will be millions and billions (an astronomical number) of variable settings to study.

Currently, there is no medical school, university, research lab, company, science foundation, or country that is able to fund and support these studies on all possible variable settings. This is why there is still no complete, systematic, and rigorous study controlling and comparing all variable settings in the simplest Chinese medicine formula.

8. Methodology of Chinese Medicine

Due to the systemic and structural differences between Chinese medicine and Western medicine, the methodology of Western medicine cannot be applied to Chinese medicine. As a result, Chinese medicine has developed its own methodology as follows.

(1) *Holistic Method*

Because the system of Chinese medicine is a multi-body, nonlinear system, all organs and systems are correlated. As a result, a holistic method is used in describing and approaching the physiological states, pathological conditions, and disease processes.

(2) *Statistical Method*

Since there is no analytical mathematics for the system of Chinese medicine yet, Chinese medicine has employed a statistical method in diagnosis and treatment procedures.

(3) *Empirical Method*

Chinese medicine originated from trial and error, practice, and experience. It has been an empirical medicine since the beginning.

(4) *Clinical Method*

Since the beginning, Chinese medicine has not used animal models. Instead, Chinese medicine is applied and tested directly on human bodies. Therefore, Chinese medicine has been a clinical medicine from the beginning.

9. Chinese Medicine vs. Complementary and Alternative Medicine (CAM)

Complementary and alternative medicine (CAM) is defined by the National Center for Complementary and Alternative Medicine (NCCAM) as follows:

> a group of diverse medical and health care systems, practices, and products that are not presently considered to be part of conventional medicine. While some scientific evidence exists regarding some CAM therapies, for most there are key questions that are yet to be answered through well-designed scientific studies — questions such as whether these therapies are safe and whether they work for the diseases or medical conditions for which they are used.

However, it is difficult to apply the definition of CAM to Chinese medicine for the following reasons.

(1) *Well-designed Scientific Studies*

In the definition of CAM, the "well-designed scientific studies" refer to randomized controlled trials (RCTs). RCTs, however, are inapplicable to the system of Chinese medicine (this issue will be further discussed later). Therefore, RCTs cannot be used as a criterion to evaluate Chinese medicine. This is the first reason that the definition of CAM cannot be applied to Chinese medicine.

(2) *Independence of CAM*

Chinese medicine has been the mainstream medicine in China and many Asian countries for hundreds and thousands of years before the existence of Western medicine and CAM. Because Western medicine was formed much later than Chinese medicine, Western medicine is an alternative medicine to Chinese medicine with respect to time sequence and from a medical history viewpoint. Therefore, it is inappropriate to regard Chinese medicine as a CAM to Western medicine.

Chinese medicine existed much earlier and independently of CAM. The efficacy and safety of Chinese medicine had been proven through thousands of years of practice. No man-made experiment can replace the thousands of years of clinical trials. This is the second reason that the definition of CAM does not apply to Chinese medicine.

10. Fundamental Characteristics of Chinese Medicine

There are many important characteristics of Chinese medicine, such as the concepts of yin-yang, five elements, meridian channels, zang xiang, jing, qi, shen, pulse, tongue, etc. However, among all these characteristics, two of them are so significant that they have answered two basic questions, and thus have been singled out and granted the status of fundamental characteristics of Chinese medicine.

Many people wonder why the two concepts are regarded as the fundamental characteristics of Chinese medicine.

The authors deem that the reasons the two concepts are regarded as fundamental characteristics of Chinese medicine are related to the following two basic questions about Chinese medicine: (1) What is Chinese medicine? (2) How does Chinese medicine work?

The two fundamental characteristics are closely associated with these two questions.

(1) *What is Chinese Medicine?*

Chinese medicine is a very large and complicated system. Rigorously speaking, a complete, detailed answer to this question would be very long.

However, if we need to answer this question succinctly, the closest answer to this question would be *holistic medicine.*

Because *holistic medicine* best describes Chinese medicine, the concept of *holism* is regarded as the first fundamental characteristic of Chinese medicine.

This fundamental characteristic differentiates Chinese medicine from Western medicine in the following ways:

(i) The concept of holism requires that Chinese medicine cannot be divided into specialties as in Western medicine.

(ii) Because of the specialty approach of Western medicine, Western medicine is a medicine of machines, in which different parts of the body are subdivided into different specialties.

(iii) Because of the holistic approach of Chinese medicine, Chinese medicine is a medicine of the human body, in which different parts are closely related.

(2) *How Does Chinese Medicine Work?*

Chinese medicine is a very complex medicine. A rigorous, complete, and detailed answer to this question would be very long.

However, if we need to answer this question succinctly, the closest answer to this question would be *treatment based on CM diagnosis.*

Because *treatment based on CM diagnosis* best describes how Chinese medicine works, it is regarded as the second fundamental characteristic of Chinese medicine.

The concept of treatment based on CM diagnosis is based on and developed from the concept of holism. However, due to its special importance, treatment based on CM diagnosis has been singled out from all other characteristics of Chinese medicine and given a position on par with the concept of holism.

The concepts of holism and treatment based on CM diagnosis are the cornerstones of Chinese medicine. These two fundamental characteristics permeate every field of Chinese medicine and differentiate it from Western medicine and other medicines. They have laid down the foundation for Chinese medicine to become a complex, dynamic, effective, and safe medicinal system.

The two fundamental characteristics of Chinese medicine have enabled Chinese medicine to endure the test of time, adapt to new challenges, and remain an outstanding medicinal system in the world for thousands of years. Holism and treatment based on CM diagnosis are the quintessence of Chinese medicine.

11. Research and Regulation of Chinese Medicine

The regulation of a medicine is based on the research of the medicine. Because the system of Chinese medicine is very different from that of Western medicine, the regulation of Chinese medicine should be different from that of Western medicine. The regulation standards of Western medicine are obtained under the single-body, nonlinear system or the multi-body, linear system, and so the conclusions drawn from the Western medical system cannot be applied directly to the multi-body, nonlinear system of Chinese medicine.

For example, the Food and Drug Administration's (FDA) standard RCTs widely used in Western medicine cannot be applied to Chinese medicine. The standards for Chinese medicine should be established within the multi-body, nonlinear system of Chinese medicine.

Another example is the heavy metal issue. This is an issue of long-term dispute between professionals in Chinese medicine and Western medicine. Many formulae in Chinese medicine contain high levels of heavy metals. According to Western medical standards, the heavy metal levels are too high in those formulae. Then someone raised the question: Are those formulae safe?

From the viewpoint of a professional in Chinese medicine, the answer is yes. Those formulae are safe as long as they are applied according to the principles and methods of Chinese medicine. These formulae have been used very safely for thousands of years in the practice of Chinese medicine. As long as those formulae are prescribed by qualified Chinese medical doctors and practitioners, they have been proven to be safe.

Chinese medicine is not a dietary supplement but a professional medicine. Most incidents relating to those heavy metal formulae were caused by unqualified practitioners of Chinese medicine. Any medicine can be dangerous if it is practiced by unqualified practitioners and Chinese medicine is no exception.

So why are these formulae with high levels of heavy metals safe in Chinese medicine? To answer this question, we need to go back to the differences between the structures of the two medical systems. In the single-body system of Western medicine, heavy metals are very toxic if above the critical threshold level. This is true when the heavy metal is in the single-body, linear system of Western medicine.

However, when the heavy metal is in a binding state in the multi-body, nonlinear system of Chinese medicine, the heavy metal's toxicity level will be changed due to the different existing state and system. As a result, the toxic threshold level of heavy metals in the multi-body, nonlinear system (e.g. restricted binding state) could become higher than the toxic threshold level of the heavy metals in the single-body, linear system (e.g. free non-binding state).

Therefore, the same heavy metal might have different toxic threshold levels in different medical systems. So it is inappropriate to apply the conclusions drawn from the single-body, linear system of Western medicine directly to the multi-body, nonlinear system of Chinese medicine.

In sum, the study and research of the efficacy and safety of Chinese herbal medicine should be carried out and conducted directly within the multi-body, nonlinear system of Chinese medicine. Conclusions drawn from studies and research within the single-body, linear system cannot be applied to Chinese medicine. Oversimplification of the multi-body, nonlinear system into a single-body, linear system will lead to inappropriate conclusions, which cannot be applied to the system of Chinese medicine.

Accordingly, regulations on Chinese medicine should be based on the studies and research conducted within the multi-body, nonlinear system of Chinese medicine. Conclusions drawn from the single-body or linear system of Western medicine should not be used to regulate Chinese medicine.

12. Nomenclature of Chinese Medicine

Chinese medicine is practiced globally. To facilitate communication among readers and practitioners in the world, it is necessary to have a consistent and standardized translation of Chinese medical terminology. It is also important to preserve intact the original meaning of the terms to ensure the efficacy and safety of Chinese medicine.

(1) *Existing Problems*

For years, many countries have been trying to establish the standard English nomenclature for Chinese medicine. However, this goal still has not been achieved. The difficulties in achieving this goal are as follows.

(i) Direct Translation

In the early years of English translations of Chinese medical texts, many terms in Chinese medicine were directly translated into Western medical terms even when there was no exact match between the two languages.

As discussed earlier, Chinese medicine and Western medicine are two completely different medicines. They are different in philosophy, fundamental characteristics, system, foundation, framework, structure, approach, principles, theory, practice, diagnosis, treatment, etc.

Because of these differences, the nomenclature and classification criteria of the two medicines are completely different. There exist very few exact matches of terms between the two medicines. As a result, many technical terms in Chinese medicine do not have exact counterparts in English. In this situation, direct translation of a Chinese medical term into an English term is inaccurate and inappropriate. It may distort the original meaning of the term in Chinese medicine, and cause misunderstandings and confusion about Chinese medicine.

Therefore, rigorously speaking, it is inappropriate to directly translate Chinese medical terms into Western medical terms.

(ii) Lack of Nomenclature Criteria and Standards

In the early years of English translations of Chinese medical texts, there were no consistent nomenclature criteria or standard. As a result, there were various translations of many Chinese medical terms. This has caused confusion about Chinese medicine.

Due to these problems, many Chinese medical terms were translated inappropriately. For example, the meaning of "xin" in Chinese medicine includes the heart, small intestine, tongue, vessels, sweat, face, gladness, bitterness, summer-heat, red, south, summer, etc. There is no one-to-one match between "xin" and "heart." However, in the past, "xin" was translated into "heart." This translation has shrunk the original meaning of "xin," and much of its original meaning has been lost or distorted. This translation does not meet the criteria of accuracy and rigorousness.

Many other terms have met similar problems as "xin." As a result, Chinese medicine has been distorted in translation and has lost its original meaning.

(2) *Criteria for Nomenclature of Chinese Medicine*

This book will use the following criteria for the nomenclature of Chinese medicine:

  (i) Accuracy: The translation of Chinese medical texts should keep the original meaning of the Chinese medical term intact. A translation deviating from this criterion may distort the original meaning in Chinese medicine.
 (ii) Rigorousness: To ensure the efficacy and safety of Chinese medicine, the translation of Chinese medical texts should be rigorous and unambiguous.
(iii) Concise: The translation of Chinese medical texts should be concise.

(3) *Standards for Nomenclature of Chinese Medicine*

This book will use the following standards for the nomenclature of Chinese medicine:

If there exists a one-to-one match between a term in Chinese medicine and a term in Western medicine, the Chinese medical term will be translated into the corresponding Western medical term.

(1) If a term in Chinese medicine does not have an exact one-to-one counterpart in Western medicine, the Chinese medical term will be given in pinyin.
(2) If a Chinese medical term is given in pinyin, the term will be defined either in the text directly or in the Glossary.

Part II

Practice

1. General Principles

Chinese medical theory was established more than 2,000 years ago. It includes a systematic, comprehensive, and complete set of diagnostic and treatment principles and methods. In this section, we will focus on Chinese medical treatments.

Generally speaking, the therapeutics of Chinese medicine can be divided into two categories: treatment principles and treatment methods.

Treatment Principles

Treatment principles are general principles directing the entire treatment procedure. Chinese medicine has a set of complete, systematic, and comprehensive treatment principles based on the philosophy and fundamental characteristics of Chinese medicine.

Concretely speaking, the treatment principles of Chinese medicine include the following:

(1) Prevention First

One branch of Chinese medicine — Chinese preventive medicine — concentrates on techniques and measurements to prevent diseases from occurring and developing. It includes the following two aspects:

(i) Prevention Before the Advent of Disease

According to Chinese medicine, all diseases have causes and roots. By removing or avoiding the causes and roots of diseases, it is possible to prevent the diseases from occurring. Chinese preventive medicine contains a set of systematic techniques and approaches to improve health by preventing diseases from occurring beforehand.

(ii) Preventing Diseases from Developing

According to Chinese medicine, once a disease has taken hold, it will evolve and develop according to its own course and pathway. By disrupting the course and pathway, Chinese preventive medicine can successfully block and prevent the disease from developing further into advanced stages. Please see the chapter on preventive medicine for more details.

(2) Searching for Essence

In Chinese medicine, a disease has two aspects: phenomena and essence. The disease may have many different phenomena. However, it is the essence that determines the disease processes. Therefore, it is important to address the essence of the disease in order to achieve better efficacy and safety.

(3) Zheng Zhi Principle

Zheng zhi is also referred to as *ni zhi*. In Chinese, *zheng* means normal, *zhi* means treatment, and *ni* means against.

The zheng zhi principle means when the disease's phenomena and essence are consistent, the treatment should be against the disease's essential and phenomenal tendency or trends. The zheng zhi principle is the allopathic treatment principle of Chinese medicine. It was established more than 1,000 years earlier than the allopathic treatment principle of Western medicine. Therefore, the zheng zhi principle of Chinese medicine probably is the world's earliest allopathic treatment principle.

(4) Fang Zhi Principle

Fang zhi is also referred to as *cong zhi*. In Chinese, *fang* means abnormal, *zhi* means treatment, and *cong* means along with.

The fang zhi principle means that when the disease's phenomena and essence are contradictory, the treatment should proceed along the essential trend or tendency of the disease. Examples of the fang zhi principle in Chinese medicine include re yin re yong, han yin han yong, sai yin sai yong, tong yin tong yong, etc. The fang zhi principle is the homeopathic treatment principle of Chinese medicine. It was established more than 2,000 years earlier than homeopathic medicine, which was started about 200 years ago. Therefore, the fang zhi principle of Chinese medicine probably is the world's earliest homeopathic treatment principle.

(5) Treating Ben

Ben is a Chinese medical term that refers to the dominant aspect of a disease process. For example, zheng qi, cause of disease, internal organs, primary disease, etc., are considered ben.

The principle of treating ben indicates that if the disease is in a relatively stabilized state or stage, it is advised to treat ben first.

(6) Treating Biao

Biao is a Chinese medical term that refers to the subordinate aspect of a disease process. For example, xie qi, symptoms, body surface, secondary diseases, etc., are considered biao.

The principle of treating biao indicates that if the disease is in an acute stage or emergent condition, it is necessary to treat biao first in order to get the disease under control as soon as possible.

(7) Treating Both Biao and Ben

In certain conditions, treating ben alone is ineffective, while treating biao alone cannot completely control the disease. In these cases, it is advised to treat both biao and ben together. This is the principle of treating both biao and ben.

(8) Strengthening Zheng

Zheng is an important term in Chinese medicine. All disease processes involve the battle between zheng and xie. If zheng overcomes xie, the patient will recover. If xie overcomes zheng, the patient will succumb. If zheng and xie reach a balanced state, the patient will be in a stage of chronic disease.

The principle of strengthening zheng is to improve zheng by means of appropriate treatment in order to help the patient move towards recovery.

(9) Eliminating Xie

Xie is a general term describing any pathogenic factors in Chinese medicine. As discussed earlier, the principle of eliminating xie is to help a patient recover by means of removing pathogenic factors as much as possible.

(10) Treating the Same Disease with Different Methods

The principle of treating the same disease with different methods means that if two patients with the same disease have different zheng, they should be treated differently. This principle is based on the fundamental characteristic of treatment based on CM diagnosis. It reflects the divergent characteristic of Chinese medicine.

(11) Treating Different Diseases with the Same Method

The principle of treating different diseases with the same method means that if two persons with different diseases have the same zheng, they will be treated with the same method. This is based on the fundamental characteristic of treatment based on CM diagnosis too. It reflects the convergent characteristic of Chinese medicine.

(12) Treatment Based on Time

According to Chinese medicine, disease processes can be greatly influenced by time, season, temporal factors, etc. The principle of treatment based on time means that the treatment should take into account time and season as factors in order to achieve the best therapeutic outcomes.

(13) Treatment Based on Location

According to Chinese medicine, disease processes vary from patient to patient by location and environment. The principle of treatment based on location means that the treatment should take into account location and environment as factors in order to achieve the optimum treatment result.

(14) Treatment Based on Individuality

Chinese medicine stresses the importance of variances of individuality between each patient in disease processes. The principle of treatment based on individuality means that each patient should be treated individually according to his/her own specific zheng. There is no one formula fitting all patients even if they have the same disease. Based on the difference in zheng, patients of the same disease will be treated differently.

Treatment Methods

Treatment methods are basic methods employed in Chinese medical treatment processes and protocols. They are more concrete methods used under the direction of treatment principles.

Treatment methods fall into two categories: general methods and specific methods.

The general methods, also called the Eight Methods, are common methods used in various aspects of Chinese medical treatments. We will discuss them in this section. Specific methods vary depending on individual zheng, disease, and case. We will discuss them in the following chapters for each individual disease.

(15) Diaphoretic Method

The diaphoretic method is to clear up the superficial xie via sweating by using appropriate herbs. For each individual case, this method will be combined with other specific methods to form the final treatment methods.

Indications: This method is applicable to the initial stage of exopathic diseases, upper body edema, the initial stage of infectious skin diseases, difficult-to-erupt measles with chills, fever, headache, body ache, thin tai, superficial pulse, etc.

Caution: Do not overuse this method.

Contraindications: This method cannot be applied to conditions when superficial xie is gone, during the eruptive stage of measles, or when there is cutaneous ulcer, spontaneous perspiration, night sweats, hemorrhage, vomiting, diarrhea, post-febrile disease, etc.

(16) Emetic Method

The emetic method is to remove xie or toxins via vomiting by using appropriate herbs.

Indications: This method is applicable to dyspepsia, stubborn tan accumulation in the upper jiao, mucus blockage of the airway, food toxins remaining in the stomach, etc.

Contraindications: This method cannot be applied to patients with advanced-stage illnesses, hemorrhage, dyspnea, or to the elderly, children, pregnant women, postpartum women, patients with qi and blood deficiency, etc.

(17) Purgative Method

The purgative method is to remove xie inside the intestinal system via inducing purgation by using appropriate herbs.

Indications: This method is applicable to accumulation of cold, heat, dryness, moisture, etc., xie inside the intestines, accumulation of fluid, dyspepsia, blood stasis, accumulation of phlegm, etc.

Contraindications: This method cannot be applied to situations when the xie is not internal, or to patients with zheng qi deficiency, menstruating women, pregnant women, seniors, patients with yang deficiency and spleen deficiency, etc.

(18) Mediation Method

The mediation method is to remove half exterior and half interior xie, and regulate the organ's qi and blood by using appropriate herbs.

Indications: Shao yang zheng, incoordination between gan and wei, gan and pi, dan and wei, chang and wei, etc.

Contraindications: Xie in the exterior, the interior, yang ming heat zheng, etc.

(19) Warming Method

The warming method is to clear cold xie and reinforce yang qi by means of appropriate herbs.

Indications: Cold invading the organs, cold due to yang deficiency, etc.

Contraindications: Yin deficiency, blood deficiency, hemorrhage, etc.

(20) Heat-clearing Method

The heat-clearing method is to remove heat xie by means of appropriate herbs.

Indications: Heat xie at qi, ying, xue when superficial xie has been removed, fever of the deficiency type, etc.

Contraindications: Non-heat-related or non-feverish conditions.

(21) Resolving Method

The resolving method is to remove or dissolve accumulated xie by means of appropriate herbs.

Indications: Masses caused by accumulation of qi, blood, foods, phlegm, moisture, fluids, etc.

Contraindications: Conditions not related to accumulation of mass.

(22) Reinforcement Method

The reinforcement method is to eliminate deficiency zheng by means of nourishing herbs.

Indications: Qi deficiency, blood deficiency, yin deficiency, yang deficiency, etc.

Contraindications: Non-deficiency conditions.

These are the general methods or Eight Methods. In practice, various methods often are jointly applied to achieve specific treatment objectives or goals.

Due to the limitations of space, the following chapters will focus mainly on Chinese herbal medicine (CHM). This, however, does not mean that other branches of Chinese medicine are inapplicable to those diseases. Other branches of Chinese medicine, such as acupuncture, tui na, an mo, tai ji, qi gong, dao yin, gua sha, all have functions for their indicated diseases.

2. Internal Medicine

Common Cold

感 冒, 伤 风

Gǎn Mào, Shāng Fēng

Definition: The common cold is characterized by a stuffy nose, running nose, headache, cough, aversion to cold, fever, body ache, etc. In Chinese medicine, it is referred to as gan mao, shang feng, etc.

Pathogenesis: The common cold is usually caused by zheng deficiency, attack on the six yin, ying wei discoordination, and failure of the lung to carry out its dispersing function.

Treatments Based on CM Diagnosis

Internal Treatments

(1) Wind Cold

Zheng: Severe aversion to cold, low fever, anhidrosis, headache, body ache, stuffy nose, heavy breathing, running nose, cough, white thin mucus, light red tongue, thin white tai, floating tight pulse.

Treatment method: Pungent warm herbs relieving the exterior, dispersing the lung and driving out cold.

Formula: Jing fang bai du san.

(2) Wind Heat

Zheng: High fever, mild aversion to wind, headache, head distension, cough, yellow thick phlegm, dry throat, red, swollen, and painful tonsil, yellow thick mucus, running nose, red tongue, thin yellow tai, floating fast pulse.

Treatment method: Pungent cool herbs relieving the exterior, dispersing the lung and clearing heat.

Formula: Yin qiao san.

(3) Summer Heat Damp

Zheng: Fever, mild aversion to wind, aching and heavy body, heavy head with distending pain, cough, thick sticky phlegm, vexation, thirst, sticky mouth, chest distress, nausea, red tongue, thin yellow greasy tai, soft fast pulse.

Treatment method: Clearing summer heat, eliminating damp, and relieving the exterior.

Formula: Xin jia xiang ru yin.

(4) Exterior Cold and Interior Heat

Zheng: Fever, aversion to cold, anhidrosis, thirst, stuffy nose, coarse voice, sore throat, cough, shortness of breath, yellow thick phlegm, constipation, yellow urine, red tongue, yellow white tai, floating fast pulse.

Treatment method: Relieving the exterior and clearing the interior, dispersing the lung and driving away wind.

Formula: Shuang jie tang.

Acupuncture Treatments

(1) Wind cold points: Feng chi, feng men, he gu, lie que, ying xiang, tai yuan, feng long, etc.

(2) Wind heat points: Da zhui, qu chi, wai guan, he gu, shao shang, etc.

Fever

发 热

Fā Rè

Definition: Fever is a symptom characterized by elevated body temperature, aversion to cold, flushing, chills, thirst, fast pulse, etc. It may exist in respiratory diseases, cardiovascular diseases, cerebrovascular diseases, hematology diseases, diabetes, cancers, etc. In Chinese medicine, it is called fa re.

Pathogenesis: Fever is usually caused by wind, cold, heat, damp, dryness, huo, toxins, etc.

Treatments Based on CM Diagnosis

Internal Treatments

(1) Defensive Energy Exterior Syndrome

Zheng: Fever, aversion to cold, stuffy nose, running nose, headache, body ache, cough, anhidrosis, dry mouth, sore throat, body heaviness, chest distress, thin white or yellow tai, floating pulse.

Treatment method: Relieving the superficial and reducing fever.

Formula: For wind cold, jing fang bai du san; for wind heat, yin qiao san.

(2) Lung Heat

Zheng: High fever, cough, gasping, yellow thick phlegm, blood in phlegm, chest pain, thirst, red tongue, yellow tai, slippery fast pulse.

Treatment method: Clearing heat and detoxifying, dispersing the lung and dissolving phlegm.

Formula: Ma xing shi gan tang.

(3) Defensive Energy Heat

Zheng: High fever, thirst, fondness for drinking, flushing, vexation, bitter taste, foul taste in the mouth, red tongue, yellow tai, strong big pulse.

Treatment method: Clearing the wei and dissolving heat.

Formula: Bai hu tang.

(4) Organ Excess

Zheng: High fever, intensifies in the afternoon, abdominal distension, constipation or fecal impaction with watery discharge, vexation, delirium, burned dry tai with prickles, deep solid powerful pulse.

Treatment method: Opening the fu and purging heat.

Formula: Da cheng qi tang.

(5) Gallbladder Heat

Zheng: Alternating fever and chills, chest and hypochondriac distension, bitter taste, dry throat, nausea, vomiting, jaundice, red tongue, yellow greasy tai, stringy fast pulse.

Treatment method: Clearing heat and soothing the dan.

Formula: Da chai hu tang.

(6) Spleen and Stomach Damp Heat

Zheng: Recessive heat, fever remains after sweating, chest and abdominal distension, anorexia, nausea, jaundice, yellow thick greasy tai, slippery fast pulse.

Treatment method: Clearing heat and inducing diuresis, promoting pi and soothing the wei.

Formula: Wang shi lian po yin.

(7) Large Intestine Damp Heat

Zheng: Fever, abdominal pain, diarrhea or dysentery, tenesmus, burning sensation around the anus, dry mouth, bitter taste, yellow urine, red tongue, yellow greasy tai, slippery fast pulse.

Treatment method: Clearing heat and inducing diuresis.

Formula: Ge gen qin lian tang.

(8) Urinary Bladder Damp Heat

Zheng: Fluctuating fever and aversion to cold, afternoon fever, urinary urgency, frequent urination, urodynia, burning sensation during urination, yellow urine, soreness in the waist or lower abdomen, red tongue, yellow greasy tai, slippery fast pulse.

Treatment method: Clearing pang guang damp heat.

Formula: Ba zheng san and xiao chai hu tang.

Dysentery

痢 疾

Lì Jí

Definition: Dysentery is characterized by abdominal pain, tenesmus, stools with blood, mucus, pus, etc. In Chinese medicine, it is called li ji.

Pathogenesis: Dysentery is usually caused by external damp heat, pathogenic toxins, inappropriate diet, etc.

Treatments Based on CM Diagnosis

Internal Treatments

(1) Damp Heat

Zheng: Abdominal pain, tenesmus, stools with blood and pus, burning sensation around the anus, little urine with yellow color, red tongue, yellow greasy tai, slippery fast pulse.

Treatment method: Clearing heat and detoxifying, regulating qi and promoting blood circulation.

Formula: Shao yao tang.

(2) Pathogenic Toxins

Zheng: Acute onset of dysentery, stools containing bright purple blood and pus, severe abdominal pain, severe tenesmus, may be accompanied by high fever, thirst, headache, dysphoria, coma, convulsion, dark red tongue, yellow dry tai, slippery fast pulse.

41

Treatment method: Clearing heat, cooling the blood, and detoxifying.

Formula: Bai tou weng tang.

(3) Cold Damp

Zheng: Abdominal pain, tenesmus, stools with plenty of jelly-like pus and little blood, anorexia, stomach distension, light red tongue, white greasy tai, soft moderate pulse.

Treatment method: Warming cold and resolving dampness.

Formula: Wei ling tang.

(4) Yin Deficiency

Zheng: Pain around the belly button, tenesmus, stools with blood and pus or sticky blood, vexation, dry mouth, red tongue, little tai, thin fast pulse.

Treatment method: Nourishing yin and cleansing the bowels.

Formula: Zhu che wan.

(5) Deficient Cold

Zheng: Dull abdominal pain, white jelly-like fluid in stools or diarrhea, anorexia, listlessness, cold limbs, soreness in the waist, aversion to cold, light red tongue, thin white tai, deep thin pulse.

Treatment method: Warming pi shen and controlling diarrhea.

Formula: Tao hua tang and zhen ren yang zang tang.

(6) Recurrent Dysentery

Zheng: Long-term on-and-off dysentery, anorexia, listlessness, abdominal pain, tenesmus, stools with pus and blood, cold limbs, aversion to cold, light red tongue, greasy tai, soft weak pulse.

Treatment method: Warming the middle jiao and cleansing the bowels, regulating qi and removing stagnation.

Formula: Lian li tang.

Acupuncture Treatments

Points: He gu, tian shu, shang ju xu, qu chi, nei ting, zhong wan, qi hai, pi shu, shen shu, guan yuan, zhong lu shu, bai hui, etc.

Malaria

疟 疾

Nuè Jí

Definition: Malaria is characterized by chills, high fever, headache, and sweating. It occurs on and off, is contagious, and may be accompanied by nausea and vomiting. It is most commonly seen in the summer and the symptoms may repeat periodically. In Chinese medicine, malaria is called nue ji.

Pathogenesis: Malaria is caused by malaria toxins, zhang du or zhang qi, etc.

Treatments Based on CM Diagnosis

Internal Treatments

(1) Common Malaria

Zheng: Starts with yawning and fatigue, followed by chills, distension in the mandible, fever, headache, flushing, thirst, sweating all over the body, then cooling down, red tongue, thin white or yellow greasy tai, stringy pulse. After one day, a similar symptom pattern repeats.

Treatment method: Driving out xie and stopping nue, resolving the superficial and the internal.

Formula: Chai hu jie nue yin.

(2) Warm Malaria

Zheng: Less chills and more fever, difficulty sweating, headache, aching bones and joints, thirst, yellow urine, constipation, red tongue, yellow tai, stringy fast pulse.

Treatment method: Clearing heat, expelling nue, and driving out xie.

Formula: Bai hu tang and gui zhi tang.

(3) Cold Malaria

Zheng: Less fever and more chills, no thirst, chest and abdominal driving out nue distension, fatigue, light red tongue, white greasy tai, stringy pulse.

Treatment method: Resolving the superficial and the internal, warming yang and driving out xie.

Formula: Chai hu gui zhi gan jiang tang.

(4) Hot Malaria

Zheng: Little or no chills, high fever, headache, aching limbs, vexation, flushing, red eyes, chest distension, nausea and vomiting, thirst, fondness for cold water, constipation, dark yellow urine, may be accompanied by coma, deep red tongue, yellow greasy or black tai, hong fast or stringy fast pulse.

Treatment method: Detoxifying and removing nue, clearing heat and protecting fluids.

Formula: Qing hao su and qing zhang tang.

(5) Cool Malaria

Zheng: More chills and little or no fever, vomiting, diarrhea, may be accompanied by coma, light tongue, white thick tai, stringy pulse.

Treatment method: Detoxifying and driving out zhang, removing dampness with aromatics.

Formula: Qing hao su and bu huan jin zheng qi san.

(6) Debilitated Malaria

Zheng: Fatigue, shortness of breath, weak voice, anorexia, pale and yellow complexion, thin with weight loss, malaria outbreak on exertion, chills and fever alternating on and off, light tongue, thin white tai, thin weak pulse.

Treatment method: Reinforcing qi and nourishing the blood, strengthening zheng and driving out xie.

Formula: He ren yin.

(7) Enlarged Malaria

Zheng: Chronic malaria with masses under the hypochondria, tenderness upon pressing, hypochondriac distension, purple tongue with ecchymosis, thin white tai, thin hesitant pulse.

Treatment method: Softening hardness and dissolving masses, removing stasis and dissolving phlegm.

Formula: Bie jia jian wan.

Cough

咳 嗽

Ké Sòu

Definition: Cough is characterized by coughing, expectoration, breathing difficulty, etc. In Chinese medicine, cough is called ke sou.

Pathogenesis: Cough is usually caused by feng, heat, huo, shi, dryness, cold, toxins, etc.

Treatments Based on CM Diagnosis

Internal Treatments

(1) Wind Cold Attacking

Zheng: Itchy throat, loud coughing, gasping, thin white tan, stuffy nose, running nose, clear nasal discharge, headache, body ache, aversion to cold, fever, anhidrosis, thin white tai, floating tight pulse.

Treatment method: Driving out feng and eliminating cold, dispersing the fei and using antitussives.

Formula: San ao tang and zhi sou san.

(2) Wind Heat Invading

Zheng: Severe coughing, gasping, hoarse voice, dry and sore throat, thick yellow phlegm, difficulty expectorating, sweating during coughing, yellow nasal discharge, thirst, headache, body ache, aversion to feng, fever, thin yellow tai, floating fast slippery pulse.

Treatment method: Driving out feng and clearing heat, dispersing the fei and using antitussives.

Formula: Sang ju yin.

(3) Wind Dryness Wounding

Zheng: Itchy throat, dry cough, choking during coughing, dry and sore throat, no or little sticky phlegm, difficulty expectorating, sputum may contain blood, dry mouth, stuffy nose, headache, aversion to cold, fever, red tongue, thin white or yellow tai, floating fast pulse.

Treatment method: Driving out feng and clearing the fei, moisturing dryness and using antitussives.

Formula: Sang xing tang.

(4) Phlegm Dampness Accumulation

Zheng: Recurrent loud coughing, chest distress especially in the morning, plenty of thick sticky phlegm which is white or grey, relief after expectoration, fatigue, abdominal distension, anorexia, diarrhea, white greasy tai, soft slippery pulse.

Treatment method: Drying dampness and dissolving phlegm, regulating qi and using antitussives.

Formula: Er chen tang and san zi yang qin tang.

(5) Phlegm Heat Accumulation

Zheng: Coughing, gasping, sound of sputum in throat, thick sticky yellow tan, difficulty expectorating, hot fishy odor, or blood in sputum, chest and hypochondriac distension, radiating pain on coughing, flushing, fever, dry sticky mouth, thirst, red tongue, thin yellow greasy tai, slippery fast pulse.

Treatment method: Clearing heat and descending the fei, dissolving tan and using antitussives.

Formula: Qing jin hua tan tang.

(6) Gan Huo Invading

Zheng: On-and-off coughing, flushing during coughing, dry throat, bitter taste, little sputum which is sticky and hard to expectorate, or sputum which is cotton-thread-like, chest and hypochondriac distension, radiating pain on coughing, fluctuating symptoms, red tongue or red tongue edge, thin yellow tai, little fluid, stringy fast pulse.

Treatment method: Clearing the gan and purging the fei, dissolving tan and using antitussives.

Formula: Dai ge san and huang qin xie bai san.

(7) Fei Yin Deficiency

Zheng: Dry cough with short sounds, blood in sputum, low fever, flushing of the zygomatic region, night sweats, dry mouth, red tongue, little tai, thin fast pulse.

Treatment method: Nourishing yin and moisturing the fei, dissolving tan and using antitussives.

Formula: Sha shen mai dong tang.

Asthma

哮 病

Xiào Bìng

Definition: Asthma is characterized by dyspnea, gasping breath, wheezing, or even the inability to lie down, etc. It occurs on and off and usually enters into the chronic stage. It has two stages: attack and remission. In Chinese medicine, asthma is called xiao bing.

Pathogenesis: Asthma is usually caused by accumulated tan inside the lung, external pathogenic factors, inappropriate diet, emotional distress, over-exertion, etc.

Treatments Based on CM Diagnosis

Internal Treatments

(A) Outbreak Stage

(1) Cold Type

Zheng: Shortness of breath, wheezing, chest distress, white thick phlegm, dark pale complexion, body cold, aversion to cold, light red tongue, white slippery tai, floating tight pulse.

Treatment method: Warming the fei and driving out cold, resolving tan and relieving wheezing.

Formula: She gan ma huang tang.

(2) Hot Type

Zheng: Heavy gasping, dyspnea, wheezing, protruding chest, hypochondriac distension, thick yellow phlegm, flushed complexion, thirst, red tongue, yellow greasy tai, slippery fast pulse.

Treatment method: Clearing heat and dispersing the fei, resolving tan and relieving wheezing.

Formula: Ding chuan tang.

(B) Remission Stage

(1) Fei Deficiency

Zheng: Shortness of breath, spontaneous perspiration, easily catching cold, occurring whenever the weather changes, light red tongue, thin white tai, weak pulse.

Treatment method: Strengthening the fei and reinforcing wei qi.

Formula: Yu ping feng san.

(2) Pi Deficiency

Zheng: Plenty of phlegm, anorexia, stomach discomfort, diarrhea, fatigue, triggered by inappropriate diet, light red tongue, white slippery tai, moderate weak pulse.

Treatment method: Strengthening the pi and resolving phlegm.

Formula: Liu jun zi tang.

(3) Shen Yang Deficiency

Zheng: Shortness of breath, gasping, wheezing, worsens with exertion, dizziness, tinnitus, soreness in the waist, weak legs, occurs after over-exertion, aversion to cold, cold limbs, pale complexion, light red tongue, white tai, deep thin pulse.

Treatment method: Nourishing shen yang.

Formula: Jin gui shen qi wan.

(4) Shen Yin Deficiency

Zheng: Shortness of breath, gasping, wheezing, worsens with exertion, dizziness, tinnitus, soreness in the waist, weak legs, occurs after over-exertion, red cheeks, dysphoria, red tongue, little tai, thin fast pulse.

Treatment method: Nourishing shen yin.

Formula: Qi wei dou qi wan.

Acupuncture Treatments

(1) Body Acupuncture

Stage of attack points: (BL13) Fei shu, (RN17) shan zhong, (Lu7) lie que, (LU5) chi ze, (BL12) feng men, (ST40) feng long, (RN22) tian tu, ding chuan, etc.

Stage of remission points: (BL13) Fei shu, (BL38) gao huang, (RN6) qi hai, (BL23) shen shu, (ST36) zu san li, (LU9) tai yuan, (KI3) tai xi, etc.

(2) Auricular Acupuncture

Points: Ping chuan, xia ping jian, fei, nao, shen men, xia jiao duan, etc.

Bronchitis

喘　证

Chuǎn Zhèng

Definition: Bronchitis is characterized by dyspnea, gasping, shortness of breath, shrugging, flaring of nares, inability to lie down, etc. It falls into two categories: excess chuan and deficiency chuan. In Chinese medicine, bronchitis is called chuan zheng.

Pathogenesis: Bronchitis is usually caused by external xie attacking the lung, tan accumulation, emotional disturbance, chronic diseases, over-exertion, etc.

Treatments Based on CM Diagnosis

Internal Treatments

(1) Feng Cold Closing the Fei

Zheng: Gasping, shortness of breath, chest distension, cough, plenty of white thin mucus, headache, stuffy nose, anhidrosis, aversion to cold, fever, light tongue, thin white slippery tai, floating tight pulse.

Treatment method: Driving out cold and dispersing the fei.

Formula: Ma huang tang.

(2) Hot Tan Suppressing the Fei

Zheng: Gasping, exhale air suddenly, chest distension and pain, plenty of thick yellow mucus which may contain blood, chest vexation, fever, sweating, thirst, fondness for cold drinks, flushing, dry throat, yellow urine, constipation, red tongue, yellow greasy tai, slippery fast pulse.

Treatment method: Clearing heat and removing mucus.

Formula: Sang bai pi tang.

(3) Tan Blocking the Fei

Zheng: Gasping, chest distension, tendency to lie supine to respire, cough, plenty of white thick mucus which is difficult to expectorate, nausea, anorexia, sticky mouth, light tongue, thick greasy white tai, slippery pulse.

Treatment method: Dissolving tan and descending qi.

Formula: Er chen tang and san zi yang qin tang.

(4) Water Attaching to the Xin and Fei

Zheng: Gasping, cough, difficulty lying down, thin and white mucus, palpitation, edema on the face and limbs, scanty urine, aversion to cold, cold extremities, purple complexion and lips, dark swollen tongue, white slippery tai, deep thin pulse.

Treatment method: Warming yang and moving water, purging blockages and suppressing gasping.

Formula: Zhen wu tang and ting li da zao xie fei tang.

(5) Gan Qi Attacking the Fei

Zheng: Dyspnea outbreak triggered by emotional disturbance, sudden shortness of breath, exhale air suddenly, distress or pain in chest, blockage in throat, insomnia, palpitation, depression, anxiety, light tongue, thin tai, stringy pulse.

Treatment method: Removing stagnation and descending qi.

Formula: Wu mo yin zi.

(6) Fei Qi Deficiency

Zheng: Gasping, shortness of breath, weak and low voice, snoring, weak coughing sound, thin mucus, spontaneous perspiration, aversion to feng, easily catching cold, light red tongue, thin white tai, weak pulse.

Treatment method: Replenishing fei qi.

Formula: Bu fei tang and yu ping feng san.

(7) Shen Qi Deficiency

Zheng: Chronic gasping, more exhaling and less inhaling, worsens on exertion, shortness of breath, urinary incontinence due to cough, blue complexion and cold limbs, light tongue, thin tai, small thin deep weak pulse.

Treatment method: Replenishing shen qi.

Formula: Jin gui shen qi wan and shen ge san.

(8) Chuan (Gasping) Exhaustion

Zheng: Severe gasping, opening the mouth for air, shrugging of shoulders, flaring of nares, inability to lie down, deterioration on exertion, palpitation, vexation, purple complexion and lips, heavy sweating, floating big pulse without root, skipping pulse or blurred pulse.

Treatment method: Reinforcing yang, stopping exhaustion, and arresting shen qi.

Formula: Shen fu tang and hei xi dan.

Bronchiectasis

肺 胀

Fèi Zhàng

Definition: Bronchiectasis is characterized by lung tissue distension by air, breathing difficulty, cough, shortness of breath, excess of phlegm, tightness in the chest, gasping, etc. In Chinese medicine, bronchiectasis is referred to as fei zhang.

Pathogenesis: Bronchiectasis is usually caused by ineffective treatments of different recurrent chronic pulmonary diseases, fei deficiency, tan accumulation, external toxins, etc.

Treatments Based on CM Diagnosis

Internal Treatments

(1) Tan Accumulation

Zheng: Cough, excess of sticky tan with white color or foam, shortness of breath, gasping, worsens on exertion, aversion to feng, easily sweating, anorexia, light red tongue, greasy tai, slippery pulse.

Treatment method: Resolving tan and descending qi, promoting the pi and enhancing the fei.

Formula: San zi yang qin tang and liu jun zi tang.

(2) Tan Heat

Zheng: Cough, excess of yellow thick phlegm which is difficult to cough out, labored breathing, vexation, chest distress, thirst, yellow urine, constipation, red tongue, yellow greasy tai, slippery fast pulse.

Treatment method: Clearing the fei and resolving phlegm, descending adverse qi and relieving gasping.

Formula: Sang bai pi tang.

(3) Tan Blocking Shen Openings

Zheng: Vague mind, delirium, vexation, sleepiness, coma, cough, gasping, sticky phlegm, tics, convulsion, dark tongue, greasy tai, slippery fast pulse.

Treatment method: Removing phlegm, cleaning the openings, and suppressing feng.

Formula: Di tan tang.

(4) Fei Shen Qi Deficiency

Zheng: Shallow breathing, shortness of breath, low voice, opening the mouth and raising the shoulders on breathing, difficulty lying down, cough, white tan full of foam, chest distress, palpitation, light dark tongue, thin tai, deep, thin, and knotted intermittent pulse.

Treatment method: Nourishing the fei and reinforcing the shen, descending qi and relieving gasping.

Formula: Ping chuan gu ben tang.

(5) Yang Deficiency and Water Inundation

Zheng: Cough, gasping, thin phlegm, edema in the face, legs, or all over the body, distended abdomen filled with water, palpitation, anorexia, little urine, purple complexion and lips, swelling dark tongue, white slippery tai, deep thin pulse.

Treatment method: Warming the shen and promoting the pi, resolving yin and diuresis.

Formula: Zhen wu tang and wu ling san.

Pulmonary Abscess

肺 痈

Fèi Yōng

Definition: Pulmonary abscess is characterized by fever, cough, chest pain, mucus which is foul-smelling and turbid and may contain blood and pus. In Chinese medicine, pulmonary abscess is referred to as fei yong.

Pathogenesis: Pulmonary abscess is usually caused by external toxins attacking the fei, hot tan accumulation, etc.

Treatments Based on CM Diagnosis

Internal Treatments

(1) Initial Stage

Zheng: Fever, mild aversion to cold, cough, sticky mucus which may contain pus, amount of mucus increases gradually, chest pain, worsens coughing, dyspnea, dry mouth and nose, light tongue, thin white or yellow tai, floating fast slippery pulse.

Treatment method: Clearing the fei and driving out xie.

Formula: Yin qiao san.

(2) Carbuncle Formation Stage

Zheng: Fever worsens, chills, followed by high fever without chills, sweating, vexation, cough, exhaling air suddenly, distension and pain in the chest, difficulty turning around, turbid yellow-greenish mucus, foul smell in the throat, dry mouth and throat, red tongue, yellow greasy tai, slippery fast pulse.

Treatment method: Clearing the fei, dissolving stasis, and removing yong.

Formula: Qian jin wei jing tang.

(3) Diabrotic Stage

Zheng: Expectoration of large amounts of mucus blended with pus and blood, which has a foul smell, or hemoptysis, chest distension and pain, gasping and inability to lie down, fever, flushing, thirst, red tongue, yellow greasy tai, hua fast or excess pulse.

Treatment method: Removing pus and detoxifying.

Formula: Jia wei jie geng tang.

(4) Recovery Stage

Zheng: Fever gradually recedes, cough reduces, amount of pus and blood in mucus reduces, foul smell reduces, mucus becomes thin and clear, mind and mood improve, appetite increases, mild chest pain, inability to lie down for long periods of time, shortness of breath, fatigue, spontaneous perspiration, night sweats, low fever, tidal fever in the afternoon, vexation, dry mouth and throat, thirst, pale complexion, weight loss, red tongue, thin tai, thin fast weak pulse.

Treatment method: Reinforcing qi, nourishing yin, and clearing heat.

Formula: Sha shen qing fei tang and zhu ye shi gao tang.

Pulmonary Tuberculosis

肺 痨

Fèi Láo

Definition: Pulmonary tuberculosis is characterized by cough, hemoptysis, hectic fever, night sweats, weight loss, etc. It is contagious. In Chinese medicine, pulmonary tuberculosis is called fei lao.

Pathogenesis: Mycobacterium tuberculosis is usually caused by lao bug and zheng qi deficiency.

Treatments Based on CM Diagnosis

Internal Treatments

(1) Fei Yin Deficiency

Zheng: Dry cough, coughing sound is short and quick, expectoration of small amounts of thick mucus which may contain blood and look red, dull pain in the chest, palms and soles hot in the afternoon, dry and hot skin, dry mouth and throat, slight night sweats, red tongue edge, thin tai, thin fast pulse.

Treatment method: Replenishing yin and nourishing the fei.

Formula: Yue hua wan.

(2) Yin Deficiency and Huo Flaming Up

Zheng: Cough, exhaling air suddenly, thick yellow mucus with blood, hemoptysis, blood is bright red, hectic fever in the afternoon, dysphoria with feverish sensation in the chest, palms, and soles, red cheeks, night sweats, thirst, vexation, insomnia, fast temper, chest pain, seminal emission in men, menopausal disorder in women, weight loss, red tongue, dry thin yellow or thin tai, thin fast pulse.

Treatment method: Nourishing yin and suppressing huo.

Formula: Bai he gu jin tang.

(3) Qi Yin Deficiency

Zheng: Weak cough, shortness of breath, low voice, thin and white mucus which may contain blood, or hemoptysis, blood is light red, hectic fever in the afternoon, aversion to feng and cold, spontaneous perspiration and night sweats, anorexia, fatigue, diarrhea, pale complexion, red cheeks, light tongue with teeth prints, thin tai, thin weak fast pulse.

Treatment method: Reinforcing qi and nourishing yin.

Formula: Bao zhen tang.

(4) Yin Yang Deficiency

Zheng: Cough, gasping, shortness of breath, white mucus which may contain blood, blood is dark, hectic fever, spontaneous perspiration, night sweats, hoarseness or loss of voice, edema of the face and limbs, palpitation, purple lips, cold limbs, aversion to cold, diarrhea, ulceration in the mouth, weight loss, spermatorrhea and impotence in men, scanty menstruation or amenia in women, light purple tongue, dry thin tai, weak thin fast or big weak pulse.

Treatment method: Nourishing yin and replenishing yang.

Formula: Bu tian da zao wan.

Pulmonary Carcinoma

肺 积

Fèi Jī

Definition: Pulmonary carcinoma is characterized by cough, hemoptysis, chest pain, fever, shortness of breath, emaciation, poor appetite, fatigue, etc. In Chinese medicine, pulmonary carcinoma is referred to as fei ji.

Pathogenesis: Pulmonary carcinoma is usually caused by toxin attacks, qi deficiency, blood deficiency, diet, emotional stress, over-exertion, etc.

Treatments Based on CM Diagnosis

Internal Treatments

(1) Qi Stagnation and Blood Stasis

Zheng: Obstructive cough, stabbing pain in the chest, pain location is fixed, chest tightness, shortness of breath, blood in mucus, blood is dark, constipation, dry mouth, dark purple lip, dark purple-red tongue with ecchymosis, thin tai, thin, hesitant, stringy pulse.

Treatment method: Moving the blood and dissolving stasis, regulating qi and removing stagnation.

Formula: Tao hong si wu tang.

(2) Tan Stasis and Accumulation

Zheng: Cough with mucus, thick mucus with white or yellow color, gasping, chest tightness and pain, dark red or purple tongue, white greasy or yellow thick tai, stringy slippery fast pulse.

Treatment method: Promoting the pi and removing shi, regulating qi and dissolving phlegm.

Formula: Er chen tang and gua lou xie bai ban xia tang.

(3) Yin Deficiency and Toxic Heat

Zheng: Cough, no or little mucus, with blood in mucus or constant hemoptysis, chest pain, vexation, insomnia, low fever with night sweats or high fever, thirst, constipation, red tongue, thin yellow tai, thin fast or big pulse.

Treatment method: Nourishing yin and clearing heat, detoxifying and removing stagnation.

Formula: Sha shen mai dong tang and wu wei xiao du yin.

(4) Qi and Yin Deficiency

Zheng: Cough, little mucus or thick mucus, low coughing sound, shortness of breath, gasping, fatigue, listlessness, pale complexion, emaciation, aversion to feng, spontaneous perspiration, night sweats, dry mouth, light red tongue, little tai, thin weak pulse.

Treatment method: Reinforcing qi and nourishing yin.

Formula: Sheng mai yin.

Coronary Heart Disease

胸 痹

Xiōng Bì

Definition: Coronary heart disease is characterized by chest pain or pain radiating to the back and shoulder, shortness of breath, gasping, difficulty lying down, etc. In Chinese medicine, coronary heart disease is referred to as xiong bi.

Pathogenesis: Coronary heart disease is usually caused by cold, inappropriate diet, stress, emotional disturbance, aging, weak constitution, etc.

Treatments Based on CM Diagnosis

Internal Treatments

(1) Xin Blood Stasis

Zheng: Stabbing pain in the chest, fixed pain location, worsens at the night, palpitation, dark purple tongue, deep hesitant pulse.

Treatment method: Promoting blood flow and resolving stasis, opening channels and relieving pain.

Formula: Xue fu zhu yu tang.

(2) Tan Accumulation

Zheng: Chest distress and pain or pain radiating to the shoulder and back, shortness of breath, gasping, heavy limbs and sluggish body, overweight, excess phlegm, light red tongue, greasy tai, slippery pulse.

Treatment method: Promoting yang and eliminating toxins, resolving tan and clearing blockages.

Formula: Gua lou xie bai ban xia tang.

(3) Yin Cold Stagnation

Zheng: Chest pain radiating to the back, worsens with cold, chest distress, shortness of breath, palpitation, gasping on exertion, pale complexion, cold limbs, light tongue, white tai, deep slow pulse.

Treatment method: Pungent warmth promoting yang, removing blockages, and dispersing cold.

Formula: Gua lou xie bai bai jiu tang.

(4) Xin Shen Yin Deficiency

Zheng: Chest distress and pain, palpitation, night sweats, vexation, insomnia, soreness in the waist and knees, tinnitus, dizziness, red tongue or with purple ecchymosis, little tai, thin fast hesitant pulse.

Treatment method: Nourishing yin and reinforcing the shen, nurturing the xin and calming the shen.

Formula: Zuo gui yin.

(5) Qi Yin Deficiency

Zheng: Dull pain and distress in the chest, on and off, palpitation, shortness of breath, listlessness, fatigue, pale complexion, dizziness, worsens on exertion, red tongue with teeth prints, thin, weak, knotted, intermittent pulse.

Treatment method: Nourishing qi and reinforcing yin, promoting blood flow and opening channels.

Formula: Sheng mai san and ren shen yang ying tang.

(6) Yang Qi Deficiency

Zheng: Chest distress, shortness of breath, pain may radiate to the back, palpitation, spontaneous sweating, aversion to cold, cold limbs, soreness in the waist and knees, pale complexion, light white or purple lips and nails, light white or purple tongue, white tai, deep thin weak pulse.

Treatment method: Nourishing qi and warming yang, promoting blood flow and opening channels.

Formula: Shen fu tang and you gui yin.

Acupuncture Treatments

(1) Body Acupuncture

Points: Shan zhong, nei guan, zu san li, jiu wei, shen men, tong li, jian shi, etc.

(2) Auricular Acupuncture

Points: Xin, shen men, pi zhi xia, jiao gan, nei fen mi, shen, wei, etc.

Irregular Heartbeat

心 悸

Xīn Jì

Definition: Irregular heartbeat is characterized by involuntary and fast beating of the heart, associated with nervousness, shortness of breath, chest tightness, dizziness, gasping, and a rapid, slow, or irregular pulse. In Chinese medicine, irregular heartbeat is referred to as xin ji.

Irregular heartbeat falls into the following two categories:

(1) Jing ji: If the palpitation is not severe, occurs only during panic attacks or tiredness, and does not happen under other conditions, the palpitation is called jing ji.
(2) Zheng chong: If the palpitation is severe, exists all the time, and gets worse during panic attacks and tiredness, it is called zheng chong.

Chronic jing ji may evolve into zheng chong.

Pathogenesis: Irregular heartbeat is usually caused by general asthenia, inappropriate diet, overwork, sexual strain, emotional factors, external pathogens, toxicosis, etc.

Treatments Based on CM Diagnosis

Internal Treatments

(1) Xin Deficiency and Dan Timidity

Zheng: Continuous palpitation, vexation, easily agitated, frightened, and scared, insomnia, excessive dreaming, poor appetite, aversion to sound, thin white tai, thin fast or thin stringy pulse.

Treatment method: Suppressing terror and resettling the will, nourishing the xin and calming the mind.

Formula: An shen ding zhi wan.

(2) Xin Pi Deficiencies

Zheng: Palpitation, shortness of breath, dizziness, pale complexion, fatigue, poor appetite, abdominal distension, diarrhea, insomnia, excessive dreaming, amnesia, light red tongue, thin weak pulse.

Treatment method: Enriching the blood and nourishing the xin, invigorating qi and calming the mind.

Formula: Gui pi tang.

(3) Yin Deficiency and Huo Hyperactivity

Zheng: Palpitation, easily scared, vexation, insomnia, dysphoria with feverish sensation in the chest, palms, and soles, dry mouth, night sweats, tinnitus, low back pain, dizziness, symptoms get worse with anxiety and strain, red and dry tongue, no or little tai, thin and fast pulse.

Treatment method: Replenishing yin and reducing huo, nourishing the xin and calming the mind.

Formula: Huang lian e jiao tang.

(4) Xin Yang Insufficiency

Zheng: Palpitation, vexation, chest tightness, shortness of breath, worsens after moving, pale complexion, cold extremities and body, light red tongue, white tai, xu, weak, deep, thin, pulse.

Treatment method: Warming and replenishing xin yang, calming the mind and resetting the will.

Formula: Gui zhi gan cao long gu mu li tang.

(5) Water Retention

Zheng: Palpitation, chest tightness and distension, thirst but no desire to drink, reduced amount of urine, edema in the lower extremities, cold extremities, dizziness, nausea, vomiting, salivation, light red tongue, slippery tai, stringy, slippery pulse or deep, thin, slippery pulse.

Treatment method: Invigorating xin yang, transforming qi, and diuresis.

Formula: Ling gui zhu gan tang.

(6) Xin Blood Stagnation

Zheng: Palpitation, chest distress, needle-like pain that occurs on and off in the heart, purple lips and nails, dark purple tongue or tongue with ecchymosis, hesitant, knotted, or intermittent pulse.

Treatment method: Promoting blood circulation by removing the stasis, and opening channels by regulating qi.

Formula: Tao ren hong hua jian.

(7) Tan Huo Disturbing the Xin

Zheng: Palpitation occurs on and off, easily occurring after a scare, chest distress and vexation, insomnia, excessive dreaming, dry mouth and bitter taste, constipation, reduced urine output, dark yellow urine, red tongue, yellow greasy tai, stringy slippery pulse.

Treatment method: Clearing heat and resolving tan, soothing the xin and calming the mind.

Formula: Huang lian wen dan tang.

Acupuncture Treatments

(1) Body Acupuncture

Points: Xi men, shen men, xin shu, ju que xue. For pi deficiency, add pi shu, zu san li, ge shu. For tan huo, add feng long, nei guan, chi ze. For water retention, add pi shu, wei shu, san yin jiao.

(2) Auricular Acupuncture

Points: Xin, nao, shen men, xiao chang, xia jiao duan.

Dizziness

眩 晕

Xuàn Yùn

Definition: Dizziness is characterized by a feeling akin to riding a boat or vehicle, rotating sensation, inability to stand, nausea, vomiting, sweating, blurred vision, pale complexion, coma, etc. In Chinese medicine, dizziness is called xuan yun.

Pathogenesis: Dizziness is usually caused by gan yin deficiency, gan yang hyperactivity, qi blood deficiency, shen jing deficiency, tan shi blockage, etc.

Treatments Based on CM Diagnosis

Internal Treatments

(1) Gan Yang Hyperactivity

Zheng: Dizziness, tinnitus, distending pain in the head, fast temper, flushing, worsens on exertion or anger, insomnia, excessive dreaming, bitter taste, red tongue, yellow tai, stringy fast pulse.

Treatment method: Suppressing the gan and lowering yang, nourishing gan shen.

Formula: Tian ma gou teng yin.

(2) Shen Yin Deficiency

Zheng: Dizziness, tinnitus, soreness in the waist and knees, listlessness, amnesia, dysphoria with warm sensation in the chest, palms, and soles, insomnia, excessive dreaming, seminal emission, red tongue, little tai, stringy thin fast pulse.

Treatment method: Nourishing shen yin and replenishing jing.

Formula: Zuo gui wan.

(3) Shen Yang Deficiency

Zheng: Dizziness, tinnitus, soreness in the waist and knees, listlessness, amnesia, cold extremities and body, aversion to cold, light red tongue, thin white tai, deep thin pulse.

Treatment method: Warming the shen and reinforcing yang.

Formula: You gui wan.

(4) Qi and Blood Deficiency

Zheng: Dizziness, triggered by exertion, pale complexion, palpitation, shortness of breath, fatigue, listlessness, anorexia, light red tongue, thin white tai, thin weak pulse.

Treatment method: Replenishing qi and nourishing the blood, promoting the pi and comforting the wei.

Formula: Gui pi tang.

(5) Tan Blockage

Zheng: Dizziness, heavy-headedness, chest distress, nausea, anorexia, excessive dreaming, light tongue, white greasy tai, soft slippery pulse.

Treatment method: Drying shi and resolving phlegm, promoting the pi and regulating middle.

Formula: Ban xia bai zhu tian ma tang.

(6) Gan Huo Flaming Up

Zheng: Vertigo, headache, red eyes, bitter taste in the mouth, distending pain in the chest and hypochondria, vexation, easily agitated, insomnia, excessive dreaming, red tongue, yellow greasy tai, stringy fast pulse.

Treatment method: Purging gan huo, clearing heat, and promoting diuresis.

Formula: Long dan xie gan tang.

(7) Blood Stasis Blockage

Zheng: Vertigo, headache, amnesia, insomnia, palpitation, depression, tinnitus, deafness, dark purple complexion and lips, ecchymosis on tongue, stringy, hesitant or thin hesitant pulse.

Treatment method: Removing stasis, opening orifices, and clearing channels.

Formula: Tong qiao huo xue tang.

Acupuncture Treatments

(1) Body Acupuncture

Points: Feng chi, bai hui, nei guan, zu san li. For gan yang hyperactivity, add tai chong, zu lin qi. For qi deficiency, add san yin jiao, pi shu, qi hai. For shen deficiency, add fu liu, qu quan. For tan blockage, add feng long, shan zhong.

(2) Auricular Acupuncture

Points: Shen, gan, pi, shen men, pi zhi xia, nei er, zhen, etc.

Stroke

中 风

Zhòng Fēng

Definition: Stroke is characterized by sudden fainting, hemiplegia, facial hemiparalysis, dysphasia, hemianesthesia, etc. In Chinese medicine, stroke is called zhong feng.

According to the depth and location of the disease, stroke is further divided into two types:

(1) Channel and collateral apoplexy: apoplexy without unconsciousness.
(2) Organ apoplexy: apoplexy with unconsciousness.

Based on the signs and symptoms, stroke is further divided into following two categories:

(1) Bi zheng: Coma, lockjaw, convulsion, etc. The signs and symptoms of yang bi include flushed complexion, feverish, fast respiration, foul-smelling mouth, restlessness, red tongue, yellow greasy tai, etc. The signs and symptoms of yin bi include pale complexion, pale lips, no movement, cold extremities, plenty of phlegm, light tongue, white greasy tai, deep slippery or slow pulse.
(2) Tuo zheng: Unconsciousness, closed eyes, opened mouth, relaxed and paralyzed limbs, cold extremities, sweating, incontinence, weak respiration, etc.

Pathogenesis: It is usually caused by inappropriate diet, asthenia, over-exertion, zheng deficiency, pathogenic attacks, etc.

Treatments Based on CM Diagnosis

Internal Treatments

(1) Feng Tan Stasis

Zheng: Hemiplegia, facial hemiparalysis, stiff tongue, dysphasia, hemianesthesia, dizziness, dim tongue, thin white or white greasy tai, stringy slippery pulse.

Treatment method: Removing stasis by promoting blood circulation, opening channels by clearing tan.

Formula: Hua tan tong luo tang.

(2) Gan Yang Hyperactivity

Zheng: Hemiplegia, hemianesthesia, stiff tongue, dysphasia, or facial hemiparalysis, dizziness, headache, flushed complexion, red eyes, bitter taste in the mouth, dry throat, vexation, yellow urine, dry stools, deep red tongue, thin yellow tai, stringy and forceful pulse.

Treatment method: Suppressing gan yang, clearing heat, and opening channels.

Formula: Tian ma gou teng yin.

(3) Tan Heat Attacking the Fu

Zheng: Hemiplegia, facial hemiparalysis, dysphasia, hemianesthesia, abdominal distension, constipation, dizziness, expectorating plenty of mucus, dim red tongue, yellow greasy tai, stringy, slippery, or big pulse.

Treatment method: Clearing tan and opening the fu organs.

Formula: Xing lou cheng qi tang.

(4) Qi Deficiency and Blood Stasis

Zheng: Hemiplegia, facial hemiparalysis, dysphasia, hemianesthesia, pale complexion, shortness of breath, fatigue, drooling, sweating, palpitation, diarrhea, edema of the extremities, dim tongue, thin white greasy tai, deep thready moderate stringy pulse.

Treatment method: Replenishing qi and promoting circulation, reinforcing zheng and clearing xie.

Formula: Bu yang huan wu tang.

(5) Yin Deficiency Leads to Feng Activation

Zheng: Hemiplegia, facial hemiparalysis, dysphasia, hemianesthesia, vexation, insomnia, dizziness, tinnitus, dysphoria with feverish sensation in the chest, palms, and soles, deep or dark red tongue, little or no tai, thin, xian, or fast pulse.

Treatment method: Nourishing gan shen, suppressing yang, and calming down feng.

Formula: Zhen gan xi feng tang.

(6) Tan Heat Blocking the Zang

Zheng: Acute onset of fainting, hemiplegia, snoring with phlegm, stiff and convulsive extremities, hot nape, back, and body, vexation, or cold hands and feet, or accompanied by hematemesis, deep red tongue, yellow, ni, or dry tai, xian, hua, fast pulse.

Treatment method: Removing heat and dissolving tan, clearing openings and restoring consciousness.

Formula: Ling yang jiao tang and an gong niu huang wan.

(7) Tan Shi Obstructing Xin Shen

Zheng: Fainting, hemiplegia, slack, weak, and cold extremities, pale complexion, dim lips, plenty of tan, dim tongue, white greasy tai, chen, slippery, or moderate pulse.

Treatment method: Reinforcing yang and clearing tan, clearing openings and restoring consciousness.

Formula: Di tan tang and su he xiang wan.

(8) Yuan Qi Collapsing

Zheng: Sudden fainting, slack and cold extremities, excessive sweating, or the whole body is cold and moist, urinary and fecal incontinence, atrophy of the tongue, dark purple tongue, white greasy tai, deep moderate pulse.

Treatment method: Replenishing qi, strengthening yang, and stopping exhaustion.

Formula: Shen fu tang.

Acupuncture Treatments

(1) Channel and Collateral Apoplexy

Upper extremity points: Jian yu, qu chi, wai guan, he gu, shou san li.

Lower extremity points: Huan tiao, yang ling quan, zu san li, kun lun, jie xi.

Facial hemiparalysis: Di cang, jia che, he gu, nei ting, tai chong, (DU26) shui gou, xia guan, (ST2) si bai, qian zheng, etc.

(2) Organ Apoplexy

Bi zheng points: Shui gou, shi er jing, tai chong, feng long, lao gong.

Trismus points: Add he gu, jia che.

Dysphasia points: Add ya men, lian quan, guan chong.

Tuo zheng points: Guan yuan, shen que (moxibustion).

Insomnia

失 眠

Shī Mián

Definition: Insomnia is characterized by sleeping disorders due to lack of nourishment or disorder of xin shen. In Chinese medicine, insomnia is called shi mian.

Pathogenesis: Insomnia is usually caused by emotional disturbance, special events, inappropriate diet, other diseases, frightening incidents, etc.

Treatments Based on CM Diagnosis

Internal Treatments

(1) Xin Huo Flaming Up

Zheng: Insomnia, vexation, restlessness, dry mouth, yellow urine, canker sores, ulceration of the tongue, red tongue tip, dry thin yellow tai, fast powerful pulse.

Treatment method: Clearing the xin and purging huo, calming the shen and tranquilizing the xin.

Formula: Zhu sha an shen wan.

(2) Gan Stagnation Huo

Zheng: Insomnia, excessive dreaming, fast temper, dizziness, head distension, red eyes, tinnitus, dry mouth, bitter taste, anorexia, constipation, yellow urine, red tongue, yellow tai, stringy fast pulse.

Treatment method: Clearing the gan and purging huo, suppressing the xin and calming the shen.

Formula: Long dan xie gan tang.

(3) Tan Heat

Zheng: Insomnia, chest tightness, vexation, nausea, eructation, heavy-headedness, dizziness, bitter taste, red tongue, yellow greasy tai, slippery fast pulse.

Treatment method: Clearing heat and resolving phlegm, soothing the middle jiao and calming the shen.

Formula: Wen dan tang.

(4) Yin Deficiency Huo

Zheng: Palpitation, vexation, restlessness, insomnia, soreness in the waist, weak feet, dizziness, tinnitus, amnesia, seminal emission, dry mouth, dysphoria with feverish sensation on the chest, palms, and soles, red tongue, little tai, thin fast pulse.

Treatment method: Nourishing yin and descending huo, clearing the xin and calming the shen.

Formula: Liu wei di huang wan and huang lian e jiao tang.

(5) Xin Pi Deficiency

Zheng: Excessive dreaming, easily awakened, palpitation, amnesia, listlessness, anorexia, dizziness, fatigue, pale complexion, may have wound or hemorrhage, light tongue, thin tai, thin weak pulse.

Treatment method: Nourishing xin pi and calming the shen.

Formula: Gui pi tang.

(6) Xin Dan Qi Deficiency

Zheng: Vexation, insomnia, excessive dreaming, easily awakened, timid, palpitation, easily frightened, shortness of breath, spontaneous perspiration, fatigue, light tongue, thin white tai, stringy thin pulse.

Treatment method: Strengthening qi and suppressing fear, calming the shen and tranquilizing zhi.

Formula: An shen ding zhi wan and suan zao ren tang.

Dementia

痴 呆

Chī Dāi

Definition: Dementia is characterized by apathy, taciturnity, slow response, amnesia, living alone, muttering, speaking incoherently, slow-wittedness, etc. In Chinese medicine, dementia is referred to as chi dai.

Pathogenesis: Dementia is usually caused by emotional stress, qi blood deficiency, shen deficiency, phlegm, stasis, etc.

Treatments Based on CM Diagnosis

Internal Treatments

(1) Sui Deficiency

Zheng: Dizziness, tinnitus, memory loss, mental capability decreases, fatigue, sleepiness, dryness of the teeth, withered hair, soreness in the waist and bone, difficulty walking, thin light tongue, thin white tai, deep thin weak pulse.

Treatment method: Strengthening the shen and nourishing the marrow, replenishing jing and reinforcing the shen.

Formula: Qi fu yin.

(2) Pi Shen Deficiency

Zheng: Apathy, taciturnity, memory loss, mental capability decreases, muttering unclearly, speaking incoherently, soreness in the waist and knees, muscle atrophy, anorexia, shortness of breath, drooling, cold limbs, abdominal pain, fondness for pressure, morning diarrhea, light white swollen tongue, white tai, little tai, deep thin weak pulse.

Treatment method: Nourishing the shen and promoting the pi, strengthening qi and producing jing.

Formula: Huan shao dan.

(3) Tan Closing Openings

Zheng: Apathy, mental function decreases, crying and laughing unexpectedly, muttering, taciturnity, slow-wittedness, anorexia, abdominal distension, excessive saliva, heavy-headedness, light tongue, white greasy tai, thin slippery pulse.

Treatment method: Promoting the pi and dissolving turbidity, removing tan and clearing openings.

Formula: Xi xin tang.

(4) Stasis Blockage

Zheng: Apathy, speaking unsmoothly, amnesia, easily frightened, abnormal thoughts, strange behavior, squamous and dry skin, dry mouth, no desire to drink, dim vision, dark tongue with ecchymosis, thin uneven pulse.

Treatment method: Moving the blood and dissolving stasis, clearing openings and awakening the mind.

Formula: Tong qiao huo xue tang.

Epilepsy

痫 病

Xián Bìng

Definition: Epilepsy is characterized by a recurrent paroxysmal mental disorder of sudden, brief attacks with falling, unconsciousness, spitting foamy saliva, upward staring eyes, convulsion, screaming, etc. In Chinese medicine, epilepsy is referred to as xian bing, xian zheng, dian xian, and yang xian feng.

Pathogenesis: Epilepsy is usually caused by emotional disturbance, inappropriate diet, genetic factors, brain trauma, etc.

Treatments Based on CM Diagnosis

Internal Treatments

(1) Feng Tan Blockage

Zheng: Sudden falling, unconsciousness, convulsion, spitting saliva, screaming, urinary and fecal incontinence, or a short period of unconsciousness and trance without convulsion, light tongue, white greasy tai, stringy slippery pulse.

Treatment method: Eliminating tan and calming feng, cleaning openings and relieving seizures.

Formula: Ding xian wan.

(2) Tan Huo Hyperactivity

Zheng: Fast temper, vexation, insomnia, thick tan which is difficult to spit out, bitter taste, dry mouth, constipation, sudden unconsciousness, convulsion, spitting saliva, screaming, red tongue, yellow greasy tai, stringy slippery fast pulse.

Treatment method: Clearing the gan and suppressing huo, resolving tan and cleaning openings.

Formula: Long dan xie gan tang and di tan tang.

(3) Xin Shen Deficiency

Zheng: Chronic recurrent epilepsy, palpitation, amnesia, dizziness, soreness in the waist and knees, listlessness, fatigue, light tongue, thin greasy tai, thin weak pulse.

Treatment method: Nourishing xin shen, promoting the pi, and resolving phlegm.

Formula: Da bu yuan jian and liu jun zi tang.

Acupuncture Treatments

Points for stage of attack: Bai hui, ren zhong, hou xi, yong quan, etc.

Points for remission stage: Jiu wei, da zhui, yao qi, jian shi, feng long, etc.

Schizophrenia

癫 病

Diān Bìng

Definition: Schizophrenia is characterized by mental depression, apathy, reticence, dementia, muttering to oneself, incoherent speech, passivity, irrational happiness, etc. In Chinese medicine, schizophrenia is referred to as dian bing.

Pathogenesis: Schizophrenia is usually caused by emotional disturbance, tan accumulation, qi stagnation, genetic factors, etc.

Treatments Based on CM Diagnosis

Internal Treatments

(1) Gan Qi Stagnation

Zheng: Mental depression, unrest, reticence, easily angered and crying, frequent deep sighs, chest and hypochondriac distress and distension, light tongue, thin white tai, stringy pulse.

Treatment method: Soothing the gan and resolving stagnation, moving qi and removing blockages.

Formula: Chai hu shu gan san.

(2) Tan Qi Stagnation

Zheng: Mental depression, apathy, reticence, dementia, speaking incoherently, muttering to oneself, irregular happiness and anger, failure to tell dirty from clean, anorexia, red tongue, white greasy tai, stringy slippery pulse.

Treatment method: Regulating qi and eliminating stagnation, dissolving tan and awakening the shen.

Formula: Shun qi dao tan tang.

(3) Xin Pi Deficiency

Zheng: In a trance, mental confusion, palpitation, easily frightened, sadness, easily crying, fatigue, anorexia, light tongue, greasy tai, deep thin weak pulse.

Treatment method: Regulating qi, enhancing the pi, and nourishing the xin.

Formula: Yang xin tang and yue ju wan.

(4) Qi Yin Deficiency

Zheng: Chronic process, in a trance, excessive talking, easily frightened, vexation, insomnia, flushing, weight loss, dry mouth, red dry tongue, little or no tai, deep thin fast pulse.

Treatment method: Reinforcing qi and nourishing yin.

Formula: Si jun zi tang and da bu yin wan.

Psychosis

狂　病

Kuáng Bìng

Definition: Psychosis is characterized by extreme excitedness, madness, cursing, damaging property, easily angered, even with the intention to injure others, etc. In Chinese medicine, psychosis is referred to as kuang bing.

Pathogenesis: Psychosis is usually caused by emotional disturbance, inappropriate diet, genetic factors, etc.

Treatments Based on CM Diagnosis

Internal Treatments

(1) Tan Huo Attacking the Shen

Zheng: Fast temper, headache, insomnia, glaring, flushing, red eyes, vexation, acute onset of madness, cursing, crying, failure to tell the difference between strangers from acquaintances, crossing walls and climbing up houses or destroying property and hurting others, not eating and sleeping, deep red tongue, yellow greasy or yellow dry tai, stringy big slippery fast pulse.

Treatment method: Clearing gan huo, eliminating phlegm, and awakening the shen.

Formula: Cheng shi sheng tie luo yin.

(2) Huo Damaging Yin

Zheng: Chronic psychosis, symptoms can be stopped, fatigue, excessive talking, easily frightened, vexation on and off, thin, flushing, dirty face, red tongue, little or no tai, thin fast pulse.

Treatment method: Nourishing yin and descending huo, soothing the shen and calming the mind.

Formula: Er yin jian.

(3) Tan Accumulation and Blood Stasis

Zheng: Chronic psychosis, dark complexion, dirty face, vexation, excessive talking, constant anger or constant singing, running away, delusion, delirium, absurd thoughts, headache, palpitation, purple dark tongue with ecchymosis, little or thin yellow tai, stringy thin hesitant pulse.

Treatment method: Removing tan and clearing stasis.

Formula: Dian kuang meng xing tang.

(4) Blood Stasis Blockage

Zheng: Insomnia, easily frightened, suspicious, delusional, speaking ambiguously, dark complexion, purple tongue with ecchymosis, thin slippery tai, small stringy or thin hesitant pulse.

Treatment method: Removing stasis and opening channels.

Formula: Ding kuang zhu yu tang.

(5) Xin Shen Disharmony

Zheng: Chronic kuang, on and off, slight recovery, delirium which can be controlled, insomnia, vexation, dry mouth, constipation, red tongue tip with fissures, no tai, thin fast pulse.

Treatment method: Nourishing yin and descending yang, maintaining communication between the xin and the shen.

Formula: Huang lian e jiao tang and hu po yang xin dan.

Gastritis

胃 痛

Wèi Tòng

Definition: Gastritis is characterized by pain around the stomach area, may be accompanied by abdominal distension, nausea, vomiting, eructation, anorexia, acid regurgitation, stomach discomfort, diarrhea, constipation, etc. In Chinese medicine, gastritis is referred to as wei tong.

Pathogenesis: Gastritis is usually caused by inappropriate diet, catching cold, emotional disturbance, pi wei deficiency, etc.

Treatments Based on CM Diagnosis

Internal Treatments

(1) Cold Attack

Zheng: Sudden stomachache, aversion to cold, relieved by warmth, worsens with cold, fondness for warm drinks, light red tongue, thin white tai, stringy tight pulse.

Treatment method: Driving out cold and relieving pain.

Formula: Liang fu wan.

(2) Food Indigestion

Zheng: Stomachache, abdominal distension, eructation with fetid odor, acid regurgitation, vomiting undigested foods, red tongue, thick greasy tai, slippery pulse.

Treatment method: Promoting digestion and removing stagnation.

Formula: Bao he wan.

(3) Gan Qi Invading the Wei

Zheng: Stomach distending pain, pain radiating to the hypochondria, frequent eructation, triggered by emotional disturbance, light red tongue, thin white tai, stringy pulse.

Treatment method: Soothing the gan and regulating qi, comforting the wei and relieving pain.

Formula: Chai hu shu gan san.

(4) Gan Wei Stagnant Heat

Zheng: Stomach heat pain, urgent pain, vexation, fast temper, acid regurgitation, gastric discomfort, dry mouth, bitter taste, red tongue, yellow tai, stringy fast pulse.

Treatment method: Clearing the gan and purging heat, regulating qi and comforting the wei.

Formula: Hua gan jian.

(5) Blood Stasis

Zheng: Stabbing pain in the stomach, pain location is fixed, refusing pressing pain worsens at night or after eating, may be accompanied by hematemesis, black stools, purple dark tongue, hesitant pulse.

Treatment method: Promoting blood circulation and removing stasis, regulating qi and relieving pain.

Formula: Shi xiao san and dan shen yin.

(6) Wei Yin Deficiency

Zheng: Dull pain in the stomach, discomfort, anorexia, dry throat and mouth, constipation, red tongue, little tai, thin fast pulse.

Treatment method: Nourishing yin and reinforcing the wei.

Formula: Yi guan jian and shao yao gan cao tang.

(7) Pi Wei Deficient Cold

Zheng: Dull pain in the stomach, fondness for warmth and pressure, worsens when hungry, relief after eating, vomiting clear fluid, listlessness, anorexia, cold limbs, diarrhea, light red tongue, white tai, deep slow weak pulse.

Treatment method: Warming the middle jiao and promoting the pi.

Formula: Huang qi jian zhong tang.

Acupuncture Treatments

(1) Body Acupuncture

Points: Zhong wan, nei guan, zu san li, qi men, yin ling quan, pi shu, wei shu, zhang men, etc.

(2) Auricular Acupuncture

Points: Wei, gan, shen men, nao, xia jiao duan, etc.

Abdominal Pain

腹 痛

Fù Tòng

Definition: Abdominal pain is characterized by pain in the abdominal area. In Chinese medicine, it is called fu tong.

Pathogenesis: Abdominal pain is usually caused by external xie, inappropriate diet, emotional disturbance, yang deficiency, etc.

Treatments Based on CM Diagnosis

Internal Treatments

(1) Cold Blockage

Zheng: Acute onset of severe abdominal pain, pain can be relieved by heat and worsens with cold, aversion to cold, cold hands and feet, dull taste, clear urine, light tongue, white greasy tai, deep tight pulse.

Treatment method: Warming the interior and dispersing cold, regulating qi and stopping pain.

Formula: Liang fu wan and zheng qi tian xiang san.

(2) Shi Heat Accumulation

Zheng: Abdominal distending pain, refusing pressure, chest distress, thirst, constipation or diarrhea, hotness, spontaneous perspiration, yellow urine, red tongue, yellow dry or greasy tai, slippery fast pulse.

Treatment method: Purging the fu and eliminating heat.

Formula: Da cheng qi tang.

(3) Middle Deficiency Zang Cold

Zheng: Abdominal pain on and off, fondness for warmth and aversion to cold, fondness for pressure during pain, worsens with hunger and exertion, relieved after eating and rest, fatigue, shortness of breath, listlessness, cold extremities, anorexia, pale complexion, diarrhea, light red tongue, thin white tai, deep thin pulse.

Treatment method: Warming the middle jiao and replenishing deficiency, relieving urgency and stopping pain.

Formula: Xiao jian zhong tang.

(4) Food Stagnation

Zheng: Abdominal distending pain, refusing pressure, eructation with fetid odor, reflux, anorexia, diarrhea, relief after defecation, stools have special foul odor, or constipation, red tongue, thick greasy tai, slippery pulse.

Treatment method: Promoting digestion and removing stagnation.

Formula: Zhi shi dao zhi wan.

(5) Qi Stagnation

Zheng: Abdominal pain, distension, and discomfort, pain radiating to the hypochondria and lower abdomen, occurs on and off, relieved after belching and flatus, worsens with worry and anger, light tongue, thin white tai, stringy pulse.

Treatment method: Soothing the gan and resolving stagnation, regulating qi and stopping pain.

Formula: Chai hu shu gan san.

(6) Blood Stasis Blockage

Zheng: Severe needle-like pain in the lower abdomen or hematuria with clots in the urine, lasts for a long time, dark purple tongue, thin white tai, thin hesitant pulse.

Treatment method: Promoting circulation and removing stasis.

Formula: Shao fu zhu yu tang.

Vomiting

呕 吐

Ǒu Tù

Definition: Vomiting is characterized by emesis and retching, either accompanied by sound or not. In Chinese medicine, it is called ou tu.

Pathogenesis: Vomiting is usually caused by external xie, inappropriate diet, emotional stress, pi wei deficiency, etc.

Treatments Based on CM Diagnosis

Internal Treatments

(1) External Xie Attacking the Wei

Zheng: Sudden vomiting, acute outbreak, fever, aversion to cold, headache, body ache, chest and stomach distension, anorexia, white tai, light red tongue, soft moderate pulse.

Treatment method: Relieving the exterior and driving out xie, soothing the wei and descending reflux.

Formula: Huo xiang zheng qi san.

(2) Food Stagnation

Zheng: Vomiting, eructation with fetid odor, stomach and abdominal distension, anorexia, worsens after eating, relieved after vomiting, diarrhea or constipation, stools with foul odor, thick greasy tai, red tongue, slippery and excess pulse.

Treatment method: Eliminating foods and resolving stagnation, soothing the wei and descending reflux.

Formula: Bao he wan.

(3) Tan Yin Retention

Zheng: Vomiting clear fluid or phlegm, chest and stomach distension, anorexia, dizziness, palpitation, borborygmus, white tai, light tongue, slippery pulse.

Treatment method: Warming and resolving tan fluid, soothing the wei, and descending reflux.

Formula: Xiao ban xia tang and ling gui zhu gan tang.

(4) Gan Qi Invading the Wei

Zheng: Vomiting, acid regurgitation, sighing, frequent belching, chest and hypochondriac distension, vexation, worsens after emotional stress, red tongue edge, thin greasy tai, stringy pulse.

Treatment method: Soothing the gan and regulating qi, soothing the wei and stopping vomiting.

Formula: Si ni san and ban xia hou po tang.

(5) Pi Wei Deficiency

Zheng: Vomiting when eating inappropriate foods, occurs on and off, poor appetite, indigestion, stomach and abdominal distension, dull mouth, lack of thirst, pale complexion, fatigue, diarrhea, light tongue, thin white tai, soft weak pulse.

Treatment method: Strengthening qi and promoting the pi, soothing the wei and descending reflux.

Formula: Xiang sha liu jun zi tang.

(6) Wei Yin Deficiency

Zheng: Recurrent vomiting, small amount of vomitus, or only vomiting saliva, or retching, dry mouth, thirst, gastric discomfort with acid regurgitation, feeling of hunger without appetite, red dry tongue, little tai, thin fast pulse.

Treatment method: Nourishing wei yin and stopping vomiting.

Formula: Mai men dong tang.

Carcinoma of the Esophagus

噎 膈

Yē Gé

Definition: Carcinoma of the esophagus may not show any symptoms in the early stage. As it progresses, it is characterized by swallowing difficulty, obstructive dysphagia, front chest pain, upper back pain, progressive emaciation, enlarged neck, hoarse voice, cough, etc. In Chinese medicine, it is called ye ge.

Pathogenesis: Carcinoma of the esophagus is usually caused by inappropriate diet, emotional stress, zang fu function disorder, etc.

Treatments Based on CM Diagnosis

Internal Treatments

(1) Tan Qi Stagnation

Zheng: Swallowing difficulty, tightness and pain in the chest and diaphragm, eructation, hiccups, vomiting, dry mouth and throat, constipation, progressive emaciation, red tongue, yellow greasy tai, deep thin slippery pulse.

Treatment method: Removing stagnation and resolving phlegm, moisturing dryness and descending qi.

Formula: Qi ge san.

(2) Jin Deficiency and Heat Accumulation

Zheng: Obstructive dysphagia with pain, difficulty swallowing solid foods, able to swallow liquids only, progressive emaciation, dry mouth and throat, constipation, dysphoria with feverish sensation in the chest, palms, and soles, red fissured tongue, dry yellow tai, stringy thin fast pulse.

Treatment method: Nourishing jin, clearing heat, and dispersing nodules.

Formula: Sha shen mai dong tang.

(3) Blood Stasis

Zheng: Obstructive dysphagia, front chest pain, vomiting sticky phlegm, dark complexion, progressive emaciation, squamous and dry skin, dark tongue with ecchymosis, greasy tai, deep hesitant pulse.

Treatment method: Removing nodules and resolving stasis, nourishing yin and supplementing blood.

Formula: Tong you tang.

(4) Yang Qi Deficiency

Zheng: Obstructive dysphagia, pale complexion, listlessness, aversion to cold, shortness of breath, vomiting saliva, facial and feet edema, abdomen distension, light red tongue, white tai, thin weak pulse.

Treatment method: Warming pi shen, reinforcing yang qi.

Formula: Bu qi yun pi tang and you gui wan.

Enteritis

泄 泻

Xiè Xiè

Definition: Enteritis is characterized by frequent defecation, stools which are fluid, watery, or contain undigested foods. In Chinese medicine, it is referred to as xie xie.

Pathogenesis: It is usually caused by external xie attack, inappropriate diet, emotional stress, pi wei deficiency, ming men huo deficiency, etc.

Treatments Based on CM Diagnosis

Internal Treatments

(1) Cold Shi

Zheng: Fluid or watery stools, abdominal pain, borborygmus, stomach distension, poor appetite, light tongue, white greasy tai, soft moderate pulse. If the patient has caught feng cold, then he will have aversion to cold, fever, headache, body ache, light tongue, thin white tai, floating pulse.

Treatment method: Removing shi by means of aromatics, relieving the exterior and dispersing cold.

Formula: Huo xiang zheng qi san.

(2) Shi Heat

Zheng: Diarrhea with urgency, abdominal pain, obstructed defecation, yellow brown stools with foul odor, burning sensation in the anus, thirst, vexation, little urine with yellow color, red tongue, yellow greasy tai, slippery fast soft pulse.

Treatment method: Clearing heat and removing shi.

Formula: Ge gen qin lian tang.

(3) Food Stagnation

Zheng: Abdominal pain, borborygmus, diarrhea with stools that smell of rotten eggs, relief after diarrhea, stomach and abdominal distension, eructation with fetid odor, anorexia, light tongue, filthy thick greasy tai, slippery pulse.

Treatment method: Eliminating food stagnation.

Formula: Bao he wan.

(4) Pi Deficiency

Zheng: Chronic diarrhea on and off, stools contain undigested foods, poor appetite, stomach discomfort after eating, defecation increases after eating greasy foods, pale yellowish complexion, fatigue, light tongue, white tai, thin weak pulse.

Treatment method: Promoting the pi and reinforcing qi.

Formula: Shen ling bai zhu san.

(5) Shen Deficiency

Zheng: Abdominal pain around the belly button area before dawn, diarrhea as soon as getting borborygmus, stools contain undigested foods, relief after defecation, aversion to cold, cold extremities, soreness in the waist and knees, light tongue, white tai, deep thin pulse.

Treatment method: Warming pi shen, stopping diarrhea with astringents.

Formula: Si shen wan.

(6) Gan Stagnation

Zheng: Chest and hypochondriac distension, belching, anorexia, abdominal pain and diarrhea after depression, anger, or emotional stress, loud borborygmus, location of pain moves, frequent flatus, light red tongue, thin white tai, stringy pulse.

Treatment method: Suppressing the gan and reinforcing the pi.

Formula: Tong xie yao fang.

Constipation

便 秘

Biàn Mì

Definition: Constipation is characterized by abnormal transmission function of the large intestine, constipation, prolonged period of defecation, dry stools, difficulty defecating, etc. In Chinese medicine, it is called bian mi.

Pathogenesis: Constipation is usually caused by heat, qi stagnation, cold, qi deficiency, yin deficiency, etc.

Treatments Based on CM Diagnosis

Internal Treatments

(1) Chang Wei Heat

Zheng: Dry stools, constipation, abdominal distending pain, flushing, hot body, dry mouth, bitter taste, vexation, yellow urine, red tongue, yellow dry tai, slippery fast pulse.

Treatment method: Purging heat and moving stagnation, moisturing the chang and catharsis.

Formula: Ma zi ren wan.

(2) Qi Stagnation

Zheng: Constipation, dry stools, difficulty defecating, intestinal sound, flatus, abdominal distension, chest and hypochondriac distension, frequent eructation, anorexia, thin greasy tai, stringy pulse.

Treatment method: Regulating qi and removing obstruction.

Formula: Liu mo tang.

(3) Yin Cold Accumulation

Zheng: Constipation, abdominal distending pain, refusing pressure, hypochodriac pain, cold limbs, eructation, vomiting, white greasy tai, stringy tight pulse.

Treatment method: Warming the interior and dispersing cold, catharsis and relieving pain.

Formula: Da huang fu zi tang.

(4) Qi Deficiency

Zheng: Having the sensation of bowel movement but difficulty defecating, stools are not dry, sweating, shortness of breath, fatigue after defecation, pale complexion, tired, light tongue, white tai, weak pulse.

Treatment method: Nourishing qi and moisturing the chang.

Formula: Huang qi tang.

(5) Blood Deficiency

Zheng: Constipation, pale complexion, palpitation, shortness of breath, insomnia, excessive dreaming, amnesia, light lips, light tongue, white tai, thin pulse.

Treatment method: Replenishing blood and moisturing dryness.

Formula: Run chang wan.

(6) Yin Deficiency

Zheng: Constipation, stools like sheep dung, emaciation, dizziness, tinnitus, flushing in the zygomatic region, vexation, insomnia, tidal fever, night sweats, soreness in the waist and knees, red tongue, little tai, thin fast pulse.

Treatment method: Nourishing yin and catharsis.

Formula: Zeng ye tang.

(7) Yang Deficiency

Zheng: Difficulty defecating, stools are dry or not dry, clear urine, pale complexion, cold limbs, cold and pain in the abdomen, relief with warmth, soreness in the waist and knees, light tongue, white tai, deep slow pulse.

Treatment method: Warming yang and catharsis.

Formula: Ji chuan jian.

Jaundice

黄　疸

Huáng Dǎn

Definition: Jaundice is characterized by yellowness of the skin, whites of the eyes, mucous membrane, and urine, etc. It falls into two categories: yang huang and yin huang. Yang huang is dominated by shi heat, and yin huang is dominated by cold shi. In Chinese medicine, it is called huang dan.

Pathogenesis: Jaundice is usually caused by seasonal pathogens, inappropriate diet, pi wei shi cold, pi wei deficiency, etc.

Treatments Based on CM Diagnosis

Internal Treatments

(A) Yang Huang

(1) Heat Dominating Shi

Zheng: Skin and whites of the eyes are bright yellow, fever, thirst, heartburn, abdominal distension, dry mouth, bitter taste, nausea, vomiting, little yellow urine, constipation, red tongue, yellow greasy tai, stringy fast pulse.

Treatment method: Clearing heat, diuresis, and purgation.

Formula: Yin chen hao tang.

(2) Shi Dominating Heat

Zheng: Skin and whites of the eyes are yellow, heavy head and body, chest and abdominal distension, anorexia, nausea and vomiting, diarrhea, yellow tongue, thick greasy light yellow tai, stringy, slippery, soft slow pulse.

Treatment method: Diuresis, resolving toxins, and clearing heat.

Formula: Yin chen wu ling san and gan lu xiao du dan.

(3) Acute Huang

Zheng: Sudden onset of jaundice, yellowness progresses rapidly, color is like gold, high fever, thirst, hypochondriac pain, abdominal distension, coma, delirium, nosebleed, hemafecia, ecchymosis on the skin, deep red tongue, yellow dry tai, stringy, slippery, thin fast pulse.

Treatment method: Clearing heat and detoxifying, cooling ying and cleaning openings.

Formula: Xi jiao san.

(B) Yin Huang

Zheng: Skin and whites of the eyes are dark yellow, anorexia, abdominal distension, loose stools, listlessness, aversion to cold, tastelessness, lack of thirst, light red tongue, greasy tai, soft slow deep pulse.

Treatment method: Promoting the pi and comforting the wei, warming cold and resolving shi.

Formula: Yin chen zhu fu tang.

Acupuncture Treatments

Yang huang points: Gan shu, yang ling quan, yin ling quan, xing jian, etc.

Yin huang points: Dan shu, pi shu, wei shu, zhong wan, guan yuan, zu san li, san yin jiao, etc.

Hepatitis

胁 痛

Xié Tòng

Definition: Hepatitis is characterized by pain in one or both sides of the hypochondria. It may be accompanied by some other symptoms. In Chinese medicine, it is referred to as xie tong.

Pathogenesis: Hepatitis is usually caused by gan qi stagnation, blood stasis, gan dan shi heat, gan yin deficiency, etc.

Treatments Based on CM Diagnosis

Internal Treatments

(1) Gan Qi Stagnation

Zheng: Hypochondriac distending pain, location of pain moves, fluctuates with emotional conditions, anorexia, eructation, light red tongue, thin tai, stringy pulse.

Treatment method: Soothing the gan and regulating qi.

Formula: Chai hu shu gan san.

(2) Blood Stasis

Zheng: Stabbing pain in the hypochondria, pain location is fixed, worsens at night, may be accompanied by nodules around the hypochondria, purple dark tongue, hesitant pulse.

Treatment method: Promoting blood circulation and removing stasis.

Formula: Fu yuan huo xue tang.

(3) Shi Heat

Zheng: Severe hypochondriac pain, refusing pressure, chest distress, anorexia, whites of the eyes are red, bitter taste, may be accompanied by jaundice, red tongue, yellow tai, stringy slippery fast pulse.

Treatment method: Clearing heat and diuresis.

Formula: Long dan xie gan tang.

(4) Gan Yin Deficiency

Zheng: Dull pain in the hypochondria, worsens on exertion, dry mouth and throat, vexation, dizziness, red tongue, little tai, stringy thin fast pulse.

Treatment method: Nourishing yin and softening the gan.

Formula: Yi guan jian.

Cholecystitis

胆　胀

Dǎn Zhàng

Definition: Cholecystitis is characterized by right hypochondrium pain due to the irregular movement of dan qi. In Chinese medicine, it is referred to as dan zhang.

Pathogenesis: Cholecystitis is usually caused by inappropriate diet, emotional stress, external xie, shi heat, over-exertion, etc.

Treatments Based on CM Diagnosis

Internal Treatments

(1) Gan Dan Qi Stagnation

Zheng: Distending pain in the right hypochondrium, pain radiating to the right shoulder, worsens with anger, chest distress, sighing, frequent belching, acid regurgitation, light tongue, white greasy tai, stringy big pulse.

Treatment method: Soothing the gan and facilitating the dan, regulating qi and promoting descending.

Formula: Chai hu shu gan san.

(2) Qi Stagnation and Blood Stasis

Zheng: Severe stabbing pain in the right hypochondrium, pain location is fixed, refusing pressure, dark complexion, dry and bitter mouth, purple tongue with ecchymosis, thin white tai, stringy thin hesitant pulse.

Treatment method: Facilitating the dan and opening channels, promoting blood movement and resolving stasis.

Formula: Si ni san and shi xiao san.

(3) Dan Stagnant Heat

Zheng: Burning pain in the right hypochondrium, bitter mouth, dry throat, flushing, red eyes, constipation, scanty urine with yellow color, vexation, insomnia, fast temper, red tongue, yellow dry thick tai, stringy fast pulse.

Treatment method: Clearing gan dan huo, removing stagnation, and stopping pain.

Formula: Qing dan tang.

(4) Gan Dan Shi Heat

Zheng: Distending pain in the right hypochondrium, chest distress, anorexia, nausea, vomiting, bitter mouth, vexation, sticky stools, jaundice, red tongue, yellow greasy tai, stringy slippery pulse.

Treatment method: Clearing heat and eliminating shi, soothing the gan and facilitating the dan.

Formula: Yin chen hao tang.

(5) Yin Deficiency Stagnation

Zheng: Vague pain in the right hypochondrium, mild burning sensation, dry mouth and throat, fast temper, vexation and hot sensation in the chest, dizziness, low fever in the afternoon, red tongue, little tai, thin fast pulse.

Treatment method: Nourishing yin and clearing heat, soothing the gan and facilitating the dan.

Formula: Yi guan jian.

(6) Yang Deficiency and Stagnation

Zheng: Distending pain in the right hypochondrium, occurs on and off, stomach and abdominal distension, vomiting clear saliva, aversion to cold, cold extremities, fatigue, shortness of breath, light red tongue, white greasy tai, stringy weak pulse.

Treatment method: Warming yang and strengthening qi, regulating the gan and facilitating the dan.

Formula: Li zhong tang.

Cirrhosis

鼓　胀

Gǔ　Zhàng

Definition: Cirrhosis is characterized by abdomen distension, pale yellow skin, protruding veins, etc. In Chinese medicine, it is referred to as gu zhang.

Pathogenesis: Cirrhosis is usually caused by emotional stress, inappropriate diet, over-exertion, toxins, jaundice, tumors, etc.

Treatments Based on CM Diagnosis

Internal Treatments

(1) Qi Stagnation and Shi Blockage

Zheng: Abdominal distension, feels soft upon palpation, hypochondriac distension or pain, anorexia, stomach distension after meals, relief after eructation, mild edema in the legs, white greasy tai, stringy thin pulse.

Treatment method: Soothing the gan and regulating qi, removing shi and dispersing distension.

Formula: Chai hu shu gan san and wei ling tang.

(2) Cold Shi Surrounding the Pi

Zheng: Abdominal enlargement, feels like water in a bag upon palpation, chest distension, slight relief with heat, tiredness and heaviness, aversion to cold, limb edema, scanty urine, diarrhea, white greasy tai, stringy slow pulse.

Treatment method: Warming yang and dispersing cold, resolving shi and awakening the pi.

Formula: Shi pi yin.

(3) Shi Heat Accumulation

Zheng: Abdominal distension, feels hard, refusing pressure, vexation, bitter taste, thirst, not wanting to drink, yellow urine, constipation or diarrhea, yellow complexion, red tongue tip and edge, yellow greasy or dark tai, stringy fast pulse.

Treatment method: Clearing heat and diuresis, purging and driving out water.

Formula: Zhong man fen xiao wan and yin chen hao tang.

(4) Gan Pi Blood Stasis

Zheng: Abdominal distension, feels hard upon palpation, protruding veins, prickly pain in the hypochondria, dark complexion, red spots around the head, neck, chest, arms, etc., purple lips, dark stools, squamous skin, dry mouth, no desire to drink water, dark purple tongue with ecchymosis, thin uneven pulse.

Treatment method: Circulating the blood and dissolving stasis, moving qi and diuresis.

Formula: Tiao ying yin.

(5) Pi Shen Yang Deficiency

Zheng: Abdominal distension, resembling a frog's abdomen, pale yellow complexion, chest distress, anorexia, diarrhea, aversion to cold, cold extremities, edema, difficulty urinating, light swollen tongue with teeth prints, thick greasy tai, deep weak pulse.

Treatment method: Warming and reinforcing pi shen, moving qi and diuresis.

Formula: Fu zi li zhong wan and wu ling san.

(6) Gan Shen Yin Deficiency

Zheng: Abdominal distension, feels hard, protruding veins, thin, dark complexion, scanty urine, thirst, dry throat, vexation, insomnia, hemorrhage from the teeth and nose, deep red tongue, little tai, stringy thin fast pulse.

Treatment method: Nourishing gan shen, cooling the blood, and resolving stasis.

Formula: Liu wei di huang wan.

(7) Gu Zhang Hemorrhage

Zheng: Abdominal distension, stomach discomfort, hemorrhage from the teeth and nose, or acute change of conditions, hematemesis, hematochezia, bright red blood or dark black stool, red tongue, yellow tai, stringy fast pulse.

Treatment method: Clearing the wei and purging huo, dissolving stasis and hemostasis.

Formula: Xie xin tang and shi hui san.

(8) Gu Zhang Coma

Zheng: Coma, high fever, vexation, anger, shouting, foul-smelling mouth, constipation, yellow scanty urine, red tongue, yellow tai, stringy fast pulse.

Treatment method: Clearing the xin and opening orifices.

Formula: An gong niu huang wan, zi xue dan, or zhi bao dan.

Hepatocarcinoma

肥 气

Féi Qì

Definition: In the early stage, hepatocarcinoma may not show any symptoms. As it progresses, it is characterized by pain in the liver area, poor appetite, stomach distension, nausea, vomiting, diarrhea, emaciation, fatigue, fever, bleeding, edema, ascites, etc. In Chinese medicine, it is referred to as ji ju.

Pathogenesis: Hepatocarcinoma is usually caused by emotional stress, diet, over-exertion, toxins, etc.

Treatments Based on CM Diagnosis

Internal Treatments

(1) Gan Qi Stagnation

Zheng: Distending pain in the right hypochondrium, chest tightness, sighing, anorexia, or diarrhea, lumps under the right hypochondrium, light red tongue, thin greasy tai, stringy pulse.

Treatment method: Soothing the gan and promoting the pi, moving the blood and dissolving stasis.

Formula: Chai hu shu gan san.

(2) Qi Stagnation and Blood Stasis

Zheng: Large masses under the right hypochondrium, pain in the liver area radiating to the back, resisting pressure, worsens at night, abdominal

112

distension, anorexia, diarrhea, listlessness, fatigue, dark tongue with ecchymosis, thin tai, deep thin stringy hesitant pulse.

Treatment method: Moving qi and circulating the blood, dissolving stasis and eliminating stagnation.

Formula: Fu yuan huo xue tang.

(3) Shi Heat Toxins

Zheng: Vexation, fast temper, jaundice, dry mouth, bitter taste, anorexia, abdominal distension, stabbing pain in the right hypochondrium, yellow urine, constipation, purple dark tongue, yellow greasy tai, stringy slippery fast pulse.

Treatment method: Clearing heat and soothing the dan, purging huo and detoxifying.

Formula: Yin chen hao tang.

(4) Gan Yin Deficiency

Zheng: Pain in the right hypochondrium, dysphoria with feverish sensation in the chest, palms, and soles, dizziness, anorexia, abdominal distension, protruding veins, hematemesis, hematochezia, subcutaneous hemorrhage, red tongue, little tai, thin fast pulse.

Treatment method: Nourishing the blood and softening the gan, cooling the blood and detoxifying.

Formula: Yi guan jian.

Glomerulonephritis

水　肿

Shuǐ Zhǒng

Definition: Glomerulonephritis is characterized by water retention in the muscle and under the skin, leading to swelling in the face, eyelids, limbs, abdomen, back, and may be accompanied by hydrothorax, ascites, etc. In Chinese medicine, it is referred to as shui zhong.

Shui zhong falls into two categories:

(1) Yang shui: exterior, hot, and excessive zheng.
(2) Yin shui: interior, deficiency, and cold zheng.

Pathogenesis: Glomerulonephritis is usually caused by external feng, water, shi, infectious toxins, and inappropriate diet, over-exertion, sexual strain, etc.

Treatments Based on CM Diagnosis

Internal Treatments

(A) Yang Shui

(1) Feng Shui

Zheng: Swelling of the eyelids, rapidly spreading to the limbs and the rest of the body, aversion to cold, fever, aching limbs and body, difficulty urinating, sore throat, light red tongue, thin white or yellow tai, floating tight slippery or fast pulse.

Treatment method: Eliminating feng and moving water.

Formula: Yue bi jia zhu tang.

(2) Shi Toxin Attack

Zheng: Swelling of the eyelids, affecting the rest of the body, difficulty urinating, skin disease, even ulcer, aversion to feng, fever, red tongue, thin yellow tai, floating fast slippery pulse.

Treatment method: Dispersing the fei and detoxifying, diuresis and reducing swelling.

Formula: Ma huang lian qiao chi xiao dou tang and wu wei xiao du yin.

(3) Water Shi Attack

Zheng: Swelling of the whole body, indentation left when pressed with a finger, scanty urine, heavy body, sleepiness, chest distress, anorexia, nausea, light red tongue, white greasy tai, deep moderate pulse.

Treatment method: Promoting the pi and resolving shi, circulating yang and diuresis.

Formula: Wu pi yin and wei ling tang.

(4) Shi Heat

Zheng: Swelling of the body, tight and shiny skin, chest distress, abdominal distension, vexation, thirst, scanty yellow urine, constipation, red tongue, yellow greasy tai, soft fast pulse.

Treatment method: Dividing and removing shi and heat.

Formula: Shu zao yin zi.

(B) Yin Shui

(1) Pi Yang Deficiency

Zheng: Swelling of the body, especially in the lower part below the waist, indentation left when pressed with a finger does not fill quickly, abdominal distension, anorexia, diarrhea, yellow complexion, listlessness, cold limbs, little urine, light red tongue, white greasy tai, deep moderate pulse.

Treatment method: Warming yang and diuresis.

Formula: Shi pi yin.

(2) Shen Yang Deficiency

Zheng: Swelling of the face and body, especially under the waist, indentation left when pressed with a finger does not fill quickly, palpitation, shortness of breath, cold, sore, and heavy waist, scanty or plenty of urine, cold limbs, aversion to cold, listlessness, pale or dark complexion, light red swollen tongue, white tai, deep thin weak pulse.

Treatment method: Warming the shen and reinforcing yang, producing qi and moving water.

Formula: Ji sheng shen qi wan and zhen wu tang.

Acupuncture Treatments

Points: Shui fen, qi hai, zu san li, san jiao shu. For yang shui, add fei shu, he gu, ren zhong. For yin shui, add pi shu, shen shu, yin ling quan.

Urinary Tract Infection

淋 证

Lìn Zhèng

Definition: Urinary tract infection is characterized by frequency of micturition, urgency of urination, dripping after urination, incomplete urination, urinary tract pain, low abdominal contracture radiating to the waist, etc. In Chinese medicine, it is referred to as lin zheng.

Pathogenesis: Urinary tract infection is usually caused by pang guang shi heat, pi shen deficiency, gan qi stagnation, etc.

Treatments Based on CM Diagnosis

Internal Treatments

(1) Heat Lin

Zheng: Scanty and frequent urination, hot stabbing pain, yellow-red urine, low abdominal contracture and distending pain, chills, fever, bitter taste, nausea, pain in the waist that refuses pressure, constipation, red tongue, yellow greasy tai, slippery fast pulse.

Treatment method: Clearing heat, diuresis, and removing lin.

Formula: Ba zheng san.

(2) Stone Lin

Zheng: Urine with sand and stone, difficulty urinating, sudden interruption of urine, pressing pain in the urinary tract, low abdominal contracture, griping pain in the waist and lower back, blood in urine, red tongue, thin

117

yellow tai, stringy fast pulse. Or pale complexion, listlessness, fatigue, light tongue with teeth prints, thin weak pulse. Or vague pain in the waist and low abdomen, hot feeling in the palms and soles, red tongue, little tai, thin fast pulse.

Treatment method: Clearing heat and diuresis, removing lin and eliminating stones.

Formula: Shi wei san.

(3) Excess Qi Lin

Zheng: Urination difficulty, pain during urination, dripping, low abdominal distending pain, thin white tai, deep stringy pulse.

Treatment method: Regulating qi and promoting circulation.

Formula: Chen xiang san.

(4) Deficient Qi Lin

Zheng: Descending and distending of the lower abdomen, dripping urine, pale complexion, light tongue, weak thin pulse.

Treatment method: Reinforcing the middle jiao and nourishing qi.

Formula: Bu zhong yi qi tang.

(5) Excess Blood Lin

Zheng: Hot and painful urination, difficulty urinating, deep red urine, may contain clots with severe pain, or vexation, yellow tai, slippery fast pulse.

Treatment method: Clearing heat and diuresis, cooling the blood and hemostasis.

Formula: Xiao ji yin zi.

(6) Deficient Blood Lin

Zheng: Light red urine, mild urination pain and difficulty, soreness in the waist and knees, listlessness, fatigue, light red tongue, thin fast pulse.

Treatment method: Nourishing yin and clearing heat, supplementing deficiency and hemostasis.

Formula: Zhi bo di huang tang.

(7) Excess Gao Lin

Zheng: Urine is cloudy like rice water, afterward looks like cotton with oil on the surface, or having clots and blood, hot pain in the urinary tract, red tongue, yellow greasy tai, empty pulse.

Treatment method: Clearing heat and diuresis, separate parts of clear and cloudy urine and excreting zhuo.

Formula: Cheng shi bi xie fen qing yin.

(8) Deficient Gao Lin

Zheng: Chronic and recurrent urination pain and difficulty, oily urine, emaciation, dizziness, fatigue, soreness in the waist and knees, light tongue, greasy tai, thin weak pulse.

Treatment method: Supplementing deficiency and removing lin.

Formula: Gao lin tang.

(9) Lao Lin

Zheng: Urine is a mild red, slight urination difficulty, occurs on and off, outbreak after exertion, soreness in the waist and knees, listlessness, fatigue, light tongue, weak pulse.

Treatment method: Promoting the pi and reinforcing the shen.

Formula: Wu bi shan yao wan.

Anuresis

癃 闭

Lóng Bì

Definition: Anuresis is characterized by a decrease in the amount of urine, urination difficulty, or complete urination blockage due to shen and pang hua disorders in bladder physiological functions. In Chinese medicine, it is referred to as long bi.

Pathogenesis: Anuresis is usually caused by shi heat, fei heat, pi qi descending, shen yuan deficiency, gan qi stagnation, urinary tract blockage, etc.

Treatments Based on CM Diagnosis

Internal Treatments

(1) Pang Guang Shi Heat

Zheng: Scanty yellow urine with hot sensation during urination, or complete blockage of urination, lower abdominal distension, bitter taste, sticky mouth, thirst but no desire to drink, constipation, red tongue, yellow greasy tai, fast pulse.

Treatment method: Clearing heat and diuresis.

Formula: Ba zheng san.

(2) Fei Heat

Zheng: Urination difficulty or complete blockage of urination, dry throat, thirst, desire to drink water, gasping, cough, red tongue, thin yellow tai, fast pulse.

Treatment method: Clearing fei heat and opening water passages.

Formula: Qing fei yin.

(3) Gan Qi Stagnation

Zheng: Urination blockage or urination difficulty, hypochondrium and lower abdominal distension, vexation, fast temper, red tongue, thin yellow tai, stringy pulse.

Treatment method: Regulating qi and diuresis.

Formula: Chen xiang san.

(4) Urinary Tract Blockage

Zheng: Urine is dripping, thread-like, or completely blocked, lower abdominal distending pain, dark purple tongue with ecchymosis, thin hesitant pulse.

Treatment method: Removing stasis and dispersing stagnation, clearing the urinary tract.

Formula: Dai di dang wan.

(5) Pi Qi Descending

Zheng: Urination difficulty or complete blockage, shortness of breath, low speech volume, lower abdominal distension, fatigue, anorexia, light tongue, thin white tai, weak pulse.

Treatment method: Ascending qing and descending zhuo, transforming qi and diuresis.

Formula: Bu zhong yi qi tang and chun ze tang.

(6) Shen Yang Deficiency

Zheng: Urination blockage, difficulty, or weakness, pale complexion, listlessness, aversion to cold, cold and weakness in the waist and knees, light tongue, white tai, deep thin weak pulse.

Treatment method: Replenishing shen yang, transforming qi, and diuresis.

Formula: Ji sheng shen qi wan.

Renal Insufficiency

关 格

Guān Gé

Definition: Renal insufficiency is characterized by uroschesis, nausea, vomiting, fatigue, headache, insomnia, chest distress, palpitation, hemorrhage, convulsion, etc. In Chinese medicine, renal insufficiency is referred to as guan ge.

Pathogenesis: Renal insufficiency is usually caused by edema, stranguria, pi shen deficiency, gan wind, shi xie, etc.

Treatments Based on CM Diagnosis

Internal Treatments

(1) Pi Shen Deficiency and Moist Heat Accumulation

Zheng: Scanty yellow urine, pale complexion, soreness in the waist and knees, fatigue, anorexia, nausea in the morning, vomiting sometimes, headache, insomnia, thin yellow greasy dry tai, thin fast soft pulse.

Treatment method: Promoting the pi and nourishing the shen, clearing heat and dissolving zhuo.

Formula: Wu bi shan yao wan and huang lian wen dan tang.

(2) Pi Shen Yang Deficiency and Cold Shi Accumulation

Zheng: Urination obstructed or scanty, clear urine, pale complexion, aversion to cold, cold legs, diarrhea, vomiting clear fluid, white slippery tai, deep thin soft pulse.

Treatment method: Warming pi shen, resolving shi, and descending zhuo.

Formula: Wen pi tang and wu zhu yu tang.

(3) Gan Shen Yin Deficiency and Gan Wind Acting Up

Zheng: Scanty urine, frequent nausea, hot flushes, gingival and nasal bleeding, dizziness, headache, limb convulsion, dark red tongue with fissures, yellow greasy or burned black dry tai, stringy thin fast pulse.

Treatment method: Nourishing gan shen, suppressing the gan, and calming wind.

Formula: Liu wei di huang wan and ling yang gou teng tang.

(4) Xie Attacking Xin Bao

Zheng: Scanty or no urine, chest distress, palpitation, chest pain, coma, carphology, delirium, nausea, vomiting, white face, dark lips, cold extremities, phlegm blockage, white greasy tai, deep hesitant pulse.

Treatment method: Eliminating phlegm and descending zhuo, using acrid warmth to clear openings.

Formula: Di tan tang and su he xiang wan.

Diabetes

消 渴

Xiāo Kě

Definition: Diabetes is characterized by frequent drinking, increased appetite, frequent urination, and gradual loss of weight. It may be accompanied by turbid urine with a sweet smell, etc. In Chinese medicine, diabetes is referred to as xiao ke.

Xiao ke is further divided into three categories:

(1) Upper xiao: mainly characterized by frequent drinking;
(2) Middle xiao: mainly characterized by increased appetite;
(3) Lower xiao: mainly characterized by frequent urination.

Pathogenesis: Diabetes is usually caused by yin deficiency, inappropriate diet, disturbed emotions, over-exertion, etc.

Treatments Based on CM Diagnosis

Internal Treatments

(1) Fei Heat and Jin Damage

Zheng: Thirst, frequent drinking, dry mouth and tongue, frequent urination, excessive urine amount, red tongue edge and tip, thin yellow tai, surging fast pulse.

Treatment method: Clearing heat and nurturing the fei, producing jin and stopping thirst.

Formula: Xiao ke fang.

124

(2) Wei Heat

Zheng: Large appetite, easily hungry, constipation, loss of weight, red tongue, yellow tai, fast powerful pulse.

Treatment method: Clearing the wei and purging huo, nourishing yin and promoting fluid.

Formula: Yu nu jian.

(3) Shen Yin Deficiency

Zheng: Frequent urination, large amount of turbid urine with a sweet smell, dry mouth and lips, red tongue, little tai, deep thin fast pulse.

Treatment method: Nourishing yin and strengthening the shen.

Formula: Liu wei di huang wan.

(4) Yin Yang Deficiency

Zheng: Frequent urination, turbid urine, urinating soon after drinking, dark complexion, dry ear helix, soreness in the waist and knees, cold body, aversion to cold, light red tongue, white tai, deep thin pulse.

Treatment method: Nourishing the shen, warming yang, and arresting discharge.

Formula: Jin gui shen qi wan.

Acupuncture Treatments

(1) Body Acupuncture

Points: Fei shu, pi shu, shen shu, zu san li, tai xi. For fei dryness, add shao shang, yu ji. For wei heat, add qu chi, nei ting, shang ju xu. For shen deficiency, add guan yuan, fu liu.

(2) Auricular Acupuncture

Points: Fei, wei, shen, mouth, san jiao, pang guang.

Abdominal Mass

症 瘕 积 聚

Zhēng Jia Jī Jù

Definition: Abdominal mass is characterized by nodules or masses in the abdomen, causing abdominal distension or pain. In Chinese medicine, it is referred to as zheng jia ji ju.

Zheng and ji have forms, and are located in the blood level. Jia and ju do not have fixed forms, and are located in the qi level.

Pathogenesis: Abdominal mass is usually caused by emotional stagnation, alcohol and food damage, cold shi attack, or is secondary to other diseases.

Treatments Based on CM Diagnosis

Internal Treatments

(A) Ju Zheng

(1) Gan Qi Stagnation

Zheng: Qi accumulates in the abdomen, attacking and traveling, occurring on and off, abdominal distending pain, discomfort in the stomach and hypochondria, light red tongue, thin white tai, stringy pulse.

Treatment method: Soothing the gan, relieving stagnation, and moving qi.

Formula: Chai hu shu gan san.

(2) Food Blockage

Zheng: Abdominal distending pain, bar-shaped protrusion from the abdomen that occurs on and off, refusing pressure, anorexia, constipation, red tongue, greasy tai, stringy slippery pulse.

Treatment method: Regulating qi, promoting digestion, and resolving phlegm.

Formula: Liu mo tang.

(B) Ji Zheng

(1) Qi Stagnation and Blood Blockage

Zheng: Soft mass in the abdomen, location fixed, distending pain, light red tongue, thin white tai, stringy pulse.

Treatment method: Regulating qi, promoting blood circulation, and opening channels.

Formula: Jin ling zi san and shi xiao san.

(2) Blood Stasis

Zheng: Hard abdominal mass, pain, location fixed, fatigue, weight loss, anorexia, dark purple tongue with ecchymosis, thin tai, thin hesitant pulse.

Treatment method: Promoting blood circulation, removing stasis, and softening the mass.

Formula: Ge xia zhu yu tang.

(3) Zheng Deficiency Stasis and Blockage

Zheng: Stone-hard mass in the abdomen, pain progresses gradually, yellow or dark complexion, thin with weight loss, anorexia, light purple tongue, little or no tai, stringy thin pulse.

Treatment method: Nourishing qi, replenishing the blood, and resolving stasis.

Formula: Ba zhen tang and hua ji wan.

Acupuncture Treatments

Ju zheng points: Zhong wan, nei guan, zu san li, tian shu, qi hai, etc.

Myodystrophy

痿 病

Wěi Bìng

Definition: Myodystrophy is characterized by limb weakness, muscle slackness and atrophy, inability to move and function normally, even paralysis, etc. In Chinese medicine, it is referred to as wei zheng.

Pathogenesis: Myodystrophy is usually caused by fei heat and jin damage, shi heat, pi wei deficiency, gan shen deficiency, etc.

Treatments Based on CM Diagnosis

Internal Treatments

(1) Fei Heat and Jin Damage

Zheng: Sudden weakness of the limbs after exterior feverish diseases, vexation, thirst, cough with little mucus, dry throat, red tongue, yellow tai, thin fast pulse.

Treatment method: Clearing heat and moistening dryness, nurturing the fei and producing jin.

Formula: Qing zao jiu fei tang.

(2) Shi Heat

Zheng: Limb weakness and atrophy, fatigue, heavy body, numbness, light edema, especially in the lower extremities, or leg heat ascending, or fever, chest distress, little yellow urine, red tongue, yellow greasy tai, soft fast pulse.

Treatment method: Clearing heat and diuresis, soothing the tendons and opening channels.

Formula: Jia wei er miao san.

(3) Pi Wei Deficiency

Zheng: Limb atrophy and weakness, progresses gradually, anorexia, diarrhea, shortness of breath, fatigue, pale complexion, light red tongue, thin white tai, thin pulse.

Treatment method: Reinforcing the pi and nourishing the wei, strengthening qi and enhancing qing.

Formula: Shen ling bai zhu san.

(4) Gan Shen Deficiency

Zheng: Slow onset of atrophy and weakness of the lower extremities, soreness in the waist and knees, inability to stand for long periods of time, dizziness, hair loss, tinnitus, seminal emission, red tongue, little tai, thin fast pulse.

Treatment method: Nourishing the gan and shen, nurturing yin, and clearing heat.

Formula: Hu qian wan.

Acupuncture Treatments

Points: (1) Upper extremities: Jian yu, qu chi, he gu, yang xi. (2) Lower extremities: Bi guan, liang qiu, zu san li, jie xi. (3) Fei heat: Chi ze, fei shu, da zhui. (4) Shi heat: Yin ling quan, pi shu. (5) Gan shen yin deficiency: Gan shu, shen shu, yang ling quan.

Acute Appendicitis

肠　痈

Cháng Yōng

Definition: Acute appendicitis is characterized by acute abdominal pain associated with other symptoms. In Chinese medicine, it is referred to as chang yong.

Pathogenesis: Acute appendicitis is usually caused by inappropriate diet, temperature discordance, walking quickly, depression, stress, etc.

Treatments Based on CM Diagnosis

Internal Treatments

(1) Initial Stage

Zheng: Abdominal pain starts at the upper abdomen or around the belly button. Then the pain migrates to the right lower abdomen. The pain type is continuous vague pain or paroxysmal colic. Pain may increase when stretching the right leg. The right lower abdomen has local tenderness or resists pressure. The lan wei xue has a pressure pain point. May be accompanied by fever, nausea, anorexia, constipation, yellow urine, red tongue, white greasy tai, stringy slippery fast pulse.

Treatment method: Moving qi and eliminating stasis, purging and clearing heat.

Formula: Da huang mu dan tang and hong teng.

(2) Purulent Stage

Zheng: Abdominal pain progresses, the right lower abdomen has strong tenderness, rebound tenderness, the abdomen skin is contracted and the tight skin, may extend to the entire abdomen. A nodule may be felt in the right lower abdomen. Continuous high fever, nausea, vomiting, anorexia, red tongue, yellow thick greasy tai, strong fast pulse.

Treatment method: Purging and clearing heat, detoxifying and expelling pus.

Formula: Da huang mu dan tang and hong teng, bai jiang cao, hua fen and zeng ye tang.

(3) Diabrotic Stage

Zheng: Abdominal pain spreads from the right lower abdomen to the entire abdomen. Abdominal skin is contracted and tight, tenderness in the entire abdomen, rebound tenderness, abdominal distension, nausea, vomiting, bowel movement frequency increases and becomes similar to that of diarrhea, urination frequency increases, may see abdominal swelling, can hear sound of water when turning the body around, sweating, squamous and dry skin, sunken eyes, dry mouth, foul-smelling mouth, red tongue, yellow thick tai, thin fast pulse.

Treatment method: Purging and eliminating pus, nourishing yin and clearing heat.

Formula: Da huang mu dan tang and zeng ye tang.

External Treatments

External application: Jin huang san, yu lu san, shuang bai san.

Enema: Da huang mu dan tang.

Acupuncture Treatments

Points: Lan wei (both sides), qu chi, nei ting, tian shu, nei guan, zhong wan, da chang shu, ci liao, etc.

3. Pediatrics

Measles
麻 疹
Má Zhěn

Definition: Measles is characterized by rash all over the body with fever, cough, running nose, watery eyes, etc. It usually occurs in children. If delayed or treated inappropriately, it may evolve into deteriorating conditions. In Chinese medicine, measles is called ma zhen.

Pathogenesis: Measles is usually caused by measles toxins attacking the fei and the pi, toxin heat invading the blood and cutaneous system.

Treatments Based on CM Diagnosis

Internal Treatments

(A) Normal Case

(1) Initial Stage

Zheng: Fever, running nose, cough, sneezing, red eyes, photophobia, watery eyes, listlessness, sleepiness. Two to three days after the fever, the mouth cavity mucosa corresponding to the cheek areas turn red, and Koplik's spots appear close to the molar teeth. Scanty urine with yellow color, diarrhea, purple dactylogram (marks on the fingers), red tongue, thin white light yellow tai, floating fast pulse.

Treatment method: Pungent cool expelling pathogens, clearing and dispersing fei qi.

Formula: Xuan du fa biao tang.

(2) Eruptive Stage

Zheng: High fever, vexation, thirst, red eyes, excessive eye secretions, photophobia, watery eyes, intensified cough, rash erupts starting from the posterior ears, neck, hairline, to the face, trunk, limbs, etc. When rash erupts in the palms, soles, and nose tip, it indicates complete eruption. Rash is small and sparsely distributed at the beginning, and the color is bright red. It gradually becomes dense and dark red, and is evenly distributed and slightly protruded. Purple dactylogram (marks on the fingers), red tongue, yellow tai, fast pulse.

Treatment method: Clearing heat, detoxifying, and assisting eruption.

Formula: Qing jie tou biao tang.

(3) Recovery Stage

Zheng: After complete eruption, rash gradually disappears orderly, fever decreases, cough reduces, energy level improves, appetite increases, skin scales shed, pigmentation, slightly yellow urine, light purple dactylogram (marks on the fingers), red tongue, little tai, thin weak pulse.

Treatment method: Nourishing yin, reinforcing qi, and detoxifying.

Formula: Sha shen mai dong tang.

(B) Abnormal Case

(1) Toxins Blocking the Fei

Zheng: Continuous high fever, severe cough, gasping, flaring of nares, thirst, dysphoria, obstructed eruption, purple dactylogram (marks on the fingers), dense and purple rash, red tongue, yellow tai, fast pulse.

Treatment method: Clearing heat and detoxifying, dispersing the fei and removing blockages.

Formula: Ma xing shi gan tang.

(2) Toxins Attacking the Throat

Zheng: Sore and swollen throat, hoarse voice, deep coughing sound, difficulty swallowing, dysphoria, purple and stagnant dactylogram (marks on the fingers), respiration difficulty, red tongue, yellow tai, fast pulse.

Treatment method: Clearing heat and detoxifying, soothing the throat and eliminating swelling.

Formula: Qing yan xia tan tang.

(3) Toxins Sunk into the Xin and Gan

Zheng: Continuous high fever, vexation, delirium, dense rash concentrated in groups all over the body, purple-red rash, purple and stagnant dactylogram (marks on the fingers), may be accompanied by coma, convulsion, purple tongue, dry yellow tai, slippery fast strong pulse.

Treatment method: Clearing the ying and detoxifying, suppressing the gan and calming feng.

Formula: Ling yang gou teng tang.

Rubella

风 痧

Fēng Shā

Definition: Rubella is characterized by fever, cough, thin sand-like rash all over the body, enlargement of the posterior ears and occipital lymph nodes, etc. In Chinese medicine, rubella is referred to as feng sha.

Pathogenesis: Rubella is usually caused by external feng heat toxins attacking fei wei and accumulating in the muscles and skin.

Treatments Based on CM Diagnosis

Internal Treatments

(1) Toxins in Fei Wei

Zheng: Fever, aversion to feng, light cough, running nose, fatigue, anorexia, light red rash, rash starts from the head and face, then spreads to the trunk and extremities, rash is evenly distributed, sparse, thin, itchy, receding after two to three days, enlargement of the posterior ears and occipital lymph nodes, purple dactylogram (marks on the fingers), red tongue, white tai, floating fast pulse.

Treatment method: Driving away feng, clearing heat, and detoxifying.

Formula: Yin qiao san.

(2) Excessive Toxin Heat

Zheng: High fever, thirst, vexation, fatigue, listlessness, crops of dense rash, bright red or purple dark rash, to the touch, severely itchy, receding slowly, yellow urine, constipation, dark purple dactylogram (marks on the fingers), red tongue, yellow tai, strong fast pulse.

Treatment method: Clearing heat, cooling the blood, and detoxifying.

Formula: Tou zhen liang jie tang.

Chickenpox

水 痘

Shuǐ Dòu

Definition: Chickenpox is characterized by fever and crops of rash developing through the stages of macules, papules, vesicles, and encrusted scabs. The rash starts in the trunk, then spreads to the head, face, and extremities. In Chinese medicine, chickenpox is referred to as shui dou.

Pathogenesis: Chickenpox is usually caused by external toxins attacking the fei and pi and accumulating in the muscles and skin.

Treatments Based on CM Diagnosis

Internal Treatments

(1) Feng Heat

Zheng: Light fever, running nose, stuffy nose, cough, sneezing, red and moist rash, clear vesicle fluid, no redness around rash, rash sparsely distributed, light itchiness, good spirits, normal bowel movement and urination, light tongue, thin white tai, floating fast pulse.

Treatment method: Driving out feng and clearing heat, detoxifying and removing moisture.

Formula: Yin qiao san.

(2) Excessive Toxin Heat

Zheng: High fever, vexation, flushed complexion, red eyes, thirst, sores in the mouth and on the tongue, dense rash, itchiness, distinct redness surrounding rash, purple and dark rash, turbid vesicle fluid, constipation, scanty yellow urine, dark red tongue, yellow dry coarse tai, strong fast pulse.

Treatment method: Clearing the ying and cooling the blood, detoxifying and resolving shi.

Formula: Qing wei jie du tang.

Fulminant Dysentery

疫 毒 痢

Yì Dú Lì

Definition: Fulminant dysentery is characterized by acute onset of high fever, coma, clonic convulsion, vomiting, abdominal pain, diarrhea, tenesmus, etc. In Chinese medicine, fulminant dysentery is referred to as yi du li.

If the gastrointestinal symptoms are not obvious, yi du li can be misdiagnosed as ordinary convulsion. Delayed or inappropriate treatment may have a fatal prognosis.

Pathogenesis: Fulminant dysentery is usually caused by contaminated foods, shi heat toxins, catching cold, hungry, fatigue, frail, etc.

Treatments Based on CM Diagnosis

Internal Treatments

(1) Toxin Blockage

Zheng: Sudden high fever, nausea, vomiting, vexation, delirium, recurrent convulsion, coma, diarrhea with pus and blood in stools. If no defecation, anal digital examination or clyster may find pus and blood in stools. Red tongue, yellow thick grey tai, slippery fast strong pulse.

Treatment method: Cleaning the intestine and detoxifying, clearing heat and inducing resuscitation.

Formula: Huang lian jie du tang.

(2) Inner Blockage and Outer Collapse

Zheng: Sudden pale or grey blue complexion, cold extremities, cold sweats, purple-red lips, patterned skin, hematemesis, breathing in short gasps, blurred vision, coma, light tongue, greasy tai, thin fast weak pulse.

Treatment method: Strengthening zheng and reversing collapse, suppressing yang and calming feng.

Formula: Shen fu long mu jiu ni tang.

Acupuncture Treatments

Points: Tian shu, zu san li, zhong wan, nei guan, qu chi, chang qiang, etc.

Ascariasis

蛔　虫　病

Huí Chóng Bìng

Definition: Ascariasis is characterized by anorexia, pale yellow complexion, on and off abdominal pain around the belly button, ascaris found in stools. In Chinese medicine, ascariasis is called hui chong bing.

Pathogenesis: Ascariasis is usually caused by ingesting foods contaminated by ascaris eggs.

Treatments Based on CM Diagnosis

Internal Treatments

(1) Common Hui

Zheng: In mild cases, slight abdominal ache around the belly button, anorexia, irregular bowel movement. In severe cases, pale yellow complexion, thin, recurrent abdominal pain, nausea, vomiting, ascaris may be found in vomit, listlessness, restlessness, teeth biting in sleep, fondness for eating mud, etc., white macules on the face, light blue macules may be seen on the sclera, small white spots on the inner side of the lower lip, red prickly spots on the tongue, ascaris in stools, red tongue, thin tai, fast pulse.

Treatment method: Eliminating ascaris and regulating the pi and wei.

Formula: Shi jun zi san.

(2) Colic Hui

Zheng: Pale yellow complexion, thin, recurrent abdominal pain, listlessness, restlessness, teeth biting in sleep, fondness for eating mud, etc., white macules on the face, light blue macules may be seen on the sclera, small white spots on the inner side of the lower lip, red prickly spots on the tongue, ascaris in stools, sudden colic around the stomach and right hypochondrium, tossing and turning, cold extremities, sweating, nausea, vomiting, ascaris can be frequently found in vomit, on and off or continuous abdominal pain, may be accompanied by fever, aversion to cold, jaundice, red tongue, yellow greasy tai, stringy fast slippery pulse.

Treatment method: Soothing ascaris, relieving pain, and eliminating ascaris.

Formula: Wu mei wan.

Acupuncture Treatments

Points: Tian shu, zhong wan, zu san li, nei guan, yang ling quan, he gu, dan shu, si bai, ying xiang, dan nang xue, ren zhong, etc.

Oxyuriasis

蛲 虫 病

Náo Chóng Bìng

Definition: Oxyuriasis is characterized by itchiness around the anus and perineum during sleep at night and restlessness. In Chinese medicine, oxyuriasis is referred to as nao chong bing.

Pathogenesis: Oxyuriasis is usually caused by ingestion of foods containing pinworm eggs.

Treatments Based on CM Diagnosis

Internal Treatment

Zheng: Itchiness around the anus and perineum, especially at night, restlessness, anorexia, vexation, yellow complexion, loss of weight, nausea, abdominal pain, frequent urination, enuresis, moist red vulva, may see pinworms moving around the anus during sleep at night.

Treatment method: Eliminating pinworms and stopping itchiness.

Formula: Qu chong fen.

External Treatment

Applying vegetable oil to the anal plica two to three times a day.

Ancylostomiasis

钩　虫　病

Gōu Chóng Bìng

Definition: Ancylostomiasis is characterized by fatigue, gasping, palpitation, yellow or pale complexion, edema, etc. In Chinese medicine, ancylostomiasis is referred to as gou chong bing.

Pathogenesis: Ancylostomiasis is usually caused by skin penetration of hookworm toxins due to bare feet or sitting on the ground, touching hookworm larvae, or ingestion of foods containing hookworm toxins.

Treatments Based on CM Diagnosis

Internal Treatment

Zheng: In the early stage the skin of the fingers and toes may be itchy, and there may be rash, redness, and swelling. Then upper abdominal pain and distension, nausea, vomiting, diarrhea, anorexia, fondness for eating sand, dust, and raw rice, etc. May be accompanied by pale and yellow complexion, dizziness, palpitation, shortness of breath, fatigue, edema, anemia, malnutrition, growth retardation, withered hair, pale lips and nails, etc.

Treatment method: Eliminating worms and regulating the pi and wei.

Formula: Quan zhong tang.

Taeniasis

绦　虫　病

Tāo Chóng Bìng

Definition: Taeniasis is characterized by anorexia, loss of weight, white segments of tapeworm in stools, etc. In Chinese medicine, taeniasis is referred to as tao chong bing.

Pathogenesis: Taeniasis is usually caused by ingesting tapeworm-contaminated beef, pork, and other foods.

Treatments Based on CM Diagnosis

Internal Treatment

Zheng: In mild cases, there may be no specific symptoms. In severe cases, yellow complexion, loss of weight, vexation, anorexia, dizziness, fatigue, chest and abdominal pain, diarrhea or anal itchiness, tapeworm segments found in stools.

Treatment method: Eliminating tapeworms and regulating the pi and wei.

Formula: Xia chong wan.

Common Cold

感 冒

Găn Mào

Definition: The common cold is characterized by acute fever, headache, sore throat, swollen and red tonsil, stuffy nose, running nose, etc. In Chinese medicine, common cold is referred to as gan mao.

Pathogenesis: Common cold is usually caused by weak organs, poor immune system, inappropriate diet, six external pathogenic factors, etc.

Treatments Based on CM Diagnosis

Internal Treatments

(1) Feng Cold

Zheng: Fever, aversion to cold, anhidrosis, headache, stuffy nose, running nose, cough, sneezing, itchy throat, floating red dactylogram (marks on the fingers), light red tongue, thin white tai, floating tight pulse.

Treatment method: Pungent warmth to expel the exterior syndrome, dispersing the fei and stopping cough.

Formula: In mild cases, cong chi tang; in severe cases, jing fang bai du san.

(2) Feng Heat

Zheng: High fever, aversion to feng, slight sweating, headache, stuffy nose, sore and red throat, running nose, thick nasal discharge, cough, sneezing, yellow and thick tan, dry mouth and thirst, purple dactylogram (marks on the fingers), red tongue, thin white or light yellow tai, floating fast pulse.

Treatment method: Pungent cool to expel the exterior syndrome, clearing heat and detoxifying.

Formula: Yin qiao san.

(3) Summer Heat

Zheng: High fever, anhidrosis or little sweating, headache, heavy body, listlessness, sleepiness, chest distress, nausea, cough, vexation, anorexia, vomiting, diarrhea, flushed complexion, red lips, purple dactylogram (marks on the fingers), red tongue, yellow tai, fast pulse.

Treatment method: Clearing summer heat and expelling the exterior syndrome, regulating the middle jiao and resolving shi.

Formula: Xin jia xiang ru yin.

(4) Epidemic

Zheng: Sudden high fever, aversion to feng and cold, sweating but fever remains, chills, body ache, listlessness, stuffy nose, running nose, cough, purple dactylogram (marks on the fingers), red tongue, thin tai, floating fast pulse.

Treatment method: Driving out feng and expelling the exterior syndrome, clearing heat and detoxifying.

Formula: Chai ge jie ji tang.

Thrush

鹅 口 疮

É Kǒu Chuāng

Definition: Thrush is characterized by cheesy white scraps all over the mouth cavity and tongue, may be accompanied by fever, refusing foods, difficulty breathing and swallowing, pale bluish complexion, rales, etc. In Chinese medicine, it is referred to as e kou chuang, also called bai kou hu, xue kou, etc.

Pathogenesis: Thrush is usually caused by genetic factors, heat in fetus, unclean mouth, infecting toxins.

Treatments Based on CM Diagnosis

Internal Treatments

(1) Xin Pi Heat

Zheng: White scraps covering the mouth cavity, cheek and tongue surface, the surrounding area is red, spreads rapidly, flushed complexion, red lips, vexation, crying, running saliva, refusing foods, yellow urine, constipation, may affect respiratory tract and esophagus causing difficulty breathing and swallowing, purple stagnant dactylogram (marks on the fingers), red tongue, yellow tai, fast pulse.

Treatment method: Clearing heat and purging the pi, eliminating huo and detoxifying.

Formula: Qing re xie pi san.

(2) Deficient Huo

Zheng: White scraps sparsely distributed in the mouth cavity and over the tongue surface, redness of the surrounding area is not obvious, or ulceration of the mouth cavity and tongue, loss of weight, pale complexion, flushing of the zygomatic region, listlessness, deficient vexation, dry mouth, lack of thirst, diarrhea, pink tongue, little tai, thin fast pulse.

Treatment method: Nourishing yin, reducing huo, and conducting huo back to its origin.

Formula: Liu wei di huang wan.

(3) Pi Deficiency and Shi Excess

Zheng: White scraps covering the mouth cavity and tongue sparsely, light color, moist, pale yellow complexion, anxiety, listlessness, diarrhea, light dactylogram (marks on the fingers), light red tongue, greasy tai, thin weak pulse.

Treatment method: Enhancing the pi and nourishing qi, regulating the wei and resolving shi.

Formula: Shen ling bai zhu san.

4. Obstetrics and Gynecology

Epimenorrhagia

月 经 先 期

Yuè Jīng Xiān Qī

Definition: Epimenorrhagia is characterized by the period beginning more than seven days earlier, existing in two consecutive menstrual cycles. It may be accompanied by profuse menstruation. In Chinese medicine, it is referred to as yue jing xian qi, also called jing zao and jing qi chao qian.

Pathogenesis: Epimenorrhagia is usually caused by heat toxins in the chong ren channels, qi deficiency, etc.

Treatments Based on CM Diagnosis

Internal Treatments

(1) Qi Deficiency

Zheng: Period starts earlier, profuse menstruation, menses is of a light color and dilute, fatigue, weakness, palpitation, shortness of breath, anorexia, diarrhea, drooping in the lower abdomen, light tongue, thin tai, thin weak pulse.

Treatment method: Nourishing qi, controlling the blood, and regulating periods.

Formula: Bu zhong yi qi tang.

(2) Excessive Heat

Zheng: Period starts earlier, profuse menstruation, menses is of a deep red color and thick and sticky, vexation, flushing, dry mouth, yellow urine, constipation, red tongue, yellow tai, fast pulse.

Treatment method: Clearing heat, cooling the blood, and regulating periods.

Formula: Qing jing san.

(3) Stasis Heat

Zheng: Period starts earlier, amount fluctuates, menses is of a purple-red color with clots, chest and hypochondriac distension, lower abdominal and breast distending pain, vexation, fast temper, bitter mouth, dry throat, red tongue, yellow thin tai, stringy fast pulse.

Treatment method: Soothing the gan, clearing heat, and regulating periods.

Formula: Dan zhi xiao yao san.

(4) Deficient Heat

Zheng: Period starts earlier, menses is of a red color and thick, flushed cheeks, dysphoria with feverish sensation in the chest, soles, and palms, tidal fever, night sweats, dry throat and mouth, vexation, insomnia, red tongue, little tai, thin fast pulse.

Treatment method: Nourishing yin, clearing heat, and regulating periods.

Formula: Liang di tang.

Acupuncture Treatments

Points: Guan yuan, qi hai, tai chong, qu chi, san yin jiao, he gu, xing jian, di ji, zu san li, pi shu, jian shi, nei guan, qi men, yin bai, etc.

Hypomenorrhea

月 经 后 期

Yuè Jīng Hòu Qī

Definition: Hypomenorrhea is characterized by a later start of the period by more than seven days, existing in two consecutive menstrual cycles. In Chinese medicine, it is referred to as yue jing hou qi, also called jing qi cuo hou and jing chi.

Pathogenesis: Hypomenorrhea is usually caused by blood deficiency, shen deficiency, blood coldness, qi stagnation, tan blockage, etc.

Treatments Based on CM Diagnosis

Internal Treatments

(1) Blood Deficiency

Zheng: Period is delayed, small amount of menses which is of a light color and dilute, lower abdominal pain, pale complexion, dim skin, dizziness, palpitation, insomnia, light lips, light tongue, white thin tai, thin weak pulse.

Treatment method: Nourishing the blood and regulating periods.

Formula: Da bu yuan jian.

(2) Shen Deficiency

Zheng: Menarche is late, period is delayed, small amount of menses which is of a light or dark color, thin, soreness in the waist and knees, frequent night urination, dizziness, tinnitus, light tongue, little moisture, thin white tai, deep slow pulse.

Treatment method: Reinforcing the shen, nourishing the blood, and regulating periods.

Formula: Zuo gui wan.

(3) Blood Coldness

Zheng: Period is delayed, small amount of menses which is of a dark color and has clots, lower abdominal cold and cramp which can be relieved with heat, pale complexion, aversion to cold, cold extremities, light or dark red tongue, thin tai, deep tight pulse.

Treatment method: Warming the channels and driving out coldness, promoting circulation and eliminating stasis.

Formula: Wen jing tang.

(4) Qi Stagnation

Zheng: Period is delayed, small amount of menses which is of a dark red color and has clots, difficulty discharging, depression, chest and hypochondriac distending pain, breast and lower abdominal distending pain, red tongue, thin tai, stringy pulse.

Treatment method: Breaking stagnation and moving qi, promoting circulation and regulating periods.

Formula: Wu yao tang.

(5) Tan Blockage

Zheng: Period delayed, small amount of menses which is of a light color, chest distress, stomach distension, anorexia, nausea, excessive phlegm, overweight, light red tongue, greasy tai, slippery pulse.

Treatment method: Drying shi and resolving phlegm, promoting circulation and regulating periods.

Formula: Er chen tang.

Acupuncture Treatments

Points: Qi hai, san yin jiao. For excessive coldness, add gui lai, tian shu. For deficient coldness, add ming men, tai xi. For blood deficiency, add zu san li, pi shu, ge shu. For qi stagnation, add li gou. For lower abdominal cold pain, add guan yuan. For palpitation and insomnia, add shen men. For lower abdominal distending pain with clots, add zhong ji, si man. May apply moxibustion.

Dysmenorrhea

痛 经

Tòng Jīng

Definition: Dysmenorrhea is characterized by lower abdominal cramps before, during, or after menstruation. It may be accompanied by other systemic symptoms such as nausea, vomiting, diarrhea, frequent urination, urgency of urination, rectal drooping, headache, dizziness, fatigue, nervousness, etc. In Chinese medicine, dysmenorrhea is referred to as tong jing, jing xing fu tong, etc.

Pathogenesis: Dysmenorrhea is usually caused by emotional trauma, change in living environment, catching cold during menstruation, etc.

Treatments Based on CM Diagnosis

Internal Treatments

(1) Qi Stagnation and Blood Stasis

Zheng: Lower abdominal cramps before or during menstruation, refusing pressure, small amount of menses, discharge is dripping and not smooth and has a dim purple color purple. If qi stagnation dominates, distending sensation overrides cramps. If blood stasis dominates, cramps override distending sensation. Clots are present and cramps decrease as clots are discharged. Purple tongue with ecchymosis, thin tai, deep stringy hesitant pulse.

Treatment method: Moving qi and promoting circulation, removing stasis and stopping cramps.

Formula: Ge xia zhu yu tang.

155

(2) Cold Shi Stagnation

Zheng: Lower abdominal cramps before or during menstruation, cramps increase on pressure and decrease with heat, small amount of menses which is dark and with clots, aversion to cold, diarrhea, light tongue, white greasy tai, deep tight pulse.

Treatment method: Warming the channels and resolving stasis, driving away cold and diuresis.

Formula: Shao fu zhu yu tang.

(3) Shi Heat Accumulation

Zheng: Lower abdominal cramps before or during menstruation, refusing pressure, burning sensation, dark red menses which is thick and has clots, distending pain in the waist or chronic lower abdominal pain that increases during menstruation, yellow urine of a small amount, red tongue, yellow greasy tai, stringy fast or soft pulse.

Treatment method: Clearing heat and resolving shi, removing stasis and stopping cramps.

Formula: Xue fu zhu yu tang.

(4) Qi Blood Deficiency

Zheng: Lower abdominal cramps during or after menstruation, fondness for pressure, small amount of menses which is of a light color, thin, pale complexion, fatigue, anorexia, diarrhea, light tongue, thin white tai, thin weak pulse.

Treatment method: Reinforcing qi and nourishing the blood, relieving spasms and cramps.

Formula: Sheng yu tang.

(5) Gan Shen Deficiency

Zheng: Lower abdominal cramps one or two days after menstruation, menses is a light or dark color and of a small amount, thin, soreness in the waist and knees, dizziness, tinnitus, tidal fever, light red tongue, thin tai, deep thin pulse.

Treatment method: Reinforcing the shen, nourishing the gan, and relieving cramps.

Formula: Tiao gan tang.

Acupuncture Treatments

(1) Body Acupuncture

Points: (i) Excessive zheng: Zhong ji, xue hai, san yin jiao, jian shi, guan yuan, qi hai, tian shu, qu quan, etc. (ii) Deficient zheng: pi shu, shen shu, qi hai, zu san li. For anorexia, add wei shu, zhong wan. For blood deficiency, add ge shu, xue hai.

(2) Auricular Acupuncture

Points: Zi gong, nei fen mi, jiao gan, shen, etc.

Menopausal Syndrome

经 断 前 后 诸 症

Jīng Duàn Qián Hòu Zhū Zhèng

Definition: Menopausal syndrome is characterized by sweating, hot flushes, dizziness, tinnitus, palpitation, insomnia, dysphoria, fast temper, tidal fever, etc., around or after menopause. In Chinese medicine, menopausal syndrome is called jing duan qian hou zhu zheng.

Pathogenesis: Menopausal syndrome is usually caused by shen deficiency, chong ren deficiency, genetic factors, changes in the environment, etc.

Treatments Based on CM Diagnosis

Internal Treatments

(1) Shen Yin Deficiency

Zheng: Dizziness, tinnitus, paroxysmal hot flushes, sweating, dysphoria with feverish sensation in the chest, palms, and soles, soreness in the waist and knees, dry skin, itchiness, dry mouth, bitter taste, constipation, urine is yellow and of a small amount, preceded menstrual cycle or indefinite menstrual cycle, menses is bright red, red tongue, little tai, thin fast pulse.

Treatment method: Nourishing shen yin and assisting shen yang.

Formula: Zuo gui yin.

(2) Shen Yang Deficiency

Zheng: Dim complexion, listlessness, cold body and extremities, soreness in the waist and knees, edema in the face and limbs, frequent night urination or urinary incontinence, large amount of menses, metrorrhagia and metrostaxis, menses color is light or dark, light tongue with swelling and teeth prints, thin white tai, deep thin weak pulse.

Treatment method: Warming the shen and reinforcing yang, warming the middle jiao and promoting the pi.

Formula: You gui wan and li zhong wan.

(3) Yin Yang Deficiency

Zheng: Aversion to cold alternates with hot flushes and sweating, dizziness, tinnitus, soreness in the waist, fatigue, red tongue, thin tai, thin pulse.

Treatment method: Nourishing the shen, reinforcing yang, and fostering the chong ren.

Formula: Er xian tang and er zhi wan.

(4) Xin Pi Deficiency

Zheng: Dysphoria, anxiety, depression, wanting to cry, insomnia, dizziness, palpitation, amnesia, anorexia, edema in the limbs, stiffness and pain in the spine and back, irregular menstruation or amenorrhea, light red tongue, thin white or thick greasy tai, thin moderate pulse.

Treatment method: Promoting the pi and nourishing qi, replenishing the blood and fostering the xin.

Formula: Gui pi tang and gan mai da zao tang.

Acupuncture Treatments

(1) Body Acupuncture

Points: Da zhui, guan yuan, qi hai, zhong wan, shen shu, he gu, zu san li, qu gu, yin tang.

(2) Auricular Acupuncture

Points: Luan chao, nei fen mi, shen men, pi zhi xia, xin, gan, pi.

Hyperemesis Gravidarum

妊 娠 恶 阻

Rèn Shēn Ě Zǔ

Definition: Hyperemesis gravidarum is characterized by protracted and pernicious nausea, vomiting, dizziness, anorexia, etc., during pregnancy. In Chinese medicine, it is called ren shen e zu.

Pathogenesis: Hyperemesis gravidarum is usually caused by chong qi going upward, failure of the wei to descend, and wei deficiency.

Treatments Based on CM Diagnosis

Internal Treatments

(1) Pi Wei Deficieincy

Zheng: Abdominal distension after pregnancy, nausea, anorexia, dull taste, vomiting thin saliva, vomiting soon after eating, fatigue, listlessness, sleepiness, light tongue, thin white tai, moderate slippery pulse.

Treatment method: Promoting the pi and regulating the wei, lowering adverse qi and stopping vomiting.

Formula: Xiang sha liu jun zi tang.

(2) Gan Wei Incoordination

Zheng: Vomiting sour or bitter water in the early stage of pregnancy, chest distension, hypochondriac pain, eructation, sighing, head distension and dizziness, dysphoria, thirst, bitter taste, red tongue, light yellow tai, stringy slippery pulse.

Treatment method: Suppressing the gan and soothing the wei, lowering adverse qi and stopping vomiting.

Formula: Su ye huang lian tang.

(3) Tan Shi Blockage

Zheng: Vomiting tan and saliva in the early stage of pregnancy, chest distension, anorexia, palpitation, shortness of breath, dull taste, greasy mouth, fatigue, light tongue, white greasy tai, slippery pulse.

Treatment method: Resolving phlegm, lowering adverse qi, and stopping vomiting.

Formula: Xiao ban xia tang and fu ling.

(4) Qi Yin Deficiency

Zheng: Severe paroxysmal vomiting after pregnancy, vomit may contain blood, listlessness, thin body, sunken eyes, fever, thirst, dry lips and tongue, red tongue, thin yellow dry tai, thin weak pulse.

Treatment method: Reinforcing qi and nourishing yin, regulating the wei and stopping vomiting.

Formula: Sheng mai san and zeng ye tang.

Acupuncture Treatments

(1) Body Acupuncture

Points: Zhong wan, nei guan, jian li, you men, zu san li, shang wan, gong sun, tai chong, etc.

(2) Auricular Acupuncture

Points: Gan, pi wei, shen men, san jiao, etc.

Threatened Abortion

胎 动 不 安

Tāi Dòng Bù Ān

Definition: Threatened abortion is characterized by small amount of bleeding, soreness in the waist, abdominal distending pain and drooping, etc., during pregnancy. These symptoms are signs of spontaneous abortion and miscarriage. It usually occurs before 18 weeks of pregnancy. In Chinese medicine, it is called tai dong bu an.

Pathogenesis: Threatened abortion is usually caused by genetic defects, deficiency and weakness of the gravida, inappropriate coitus, other diseases the gravida contracts after pregnancy, injury, surgery, medication the gravida takes, etc.

Treatments Based on CM Diagnosis

Internal Treatments

(1) Shen Deficiency

Zheng: Small amount of bleeding during pregnancy, blood is a light red color and thin or a dark color like black bean soup, soreness and drooping of the waist and lower abdomen, dizziness, tinnitus, soreness and weakness of the legs, frequent urination or urinary incontinence, or the gravida has a history of abortion and miscarriage, light tongue, white tai, deep weak pulse.

Treatment method: Strengthening the shen, soothing the fetus, and reinforcing qi.

Formula: Shou tai wan.

(2) Qi Deficiency

Zheng: Frequent bleeding during pregnancy, blood is a light red color, thin, abdominal distension, soreness in the waist, drooping of the lower abdomen, pale complexion, listlessness, or bleeding may increase, which may indicate spontaneous abortion, light red tongue, thin tai, deep weak pulse.

Treatment method: Replenishing qi and nourishing the blood, strengthening and soothing the fetus.

Formula: Ju yuan jian.

(3) Blood Deficiency

Zheng: Small amount of bleeding during pregnancy, blood is a light red color, thin, soreness in the waist, pale yellow complexion, fatigue, dim skin color, light red tongue, thin white tai, thin slippery pulse.

Treatment method: Nourishing the blood, reinforcing qi, and soothing the fetus.

Formula: Tai yuan yin.

(4) Blood Heat

Zheng: Bleeding during pregnancy, blood is a bright red color, soreness and distension in the waist and lower abdomen, dysphoria with feverish sensation on the chest, palms, and soles, dry mouth and throat, tidal fever, scanty urine with yellow color, constipation, red tongue, yellow dry tai, slippery stringy fast pulse.

Treatment method: Nourishing yin and clearing heat, replenishing the blood and soothing the fetus.

Formula: Bao yin jian.

(5) Trauma

Zheng: The gravida experiences physical trauma during pregnancy, soreness in the waist, drooping of the lower abdomen, or bleeding, red tongue, thin white tai, slippery weak pulse.

Treatment method: Regulating qi and nourishing the blood, soothing and protecting the fetus.

Formula: Sheng yu tang.

Retarded Growth of the Fetus

胎 萎 不 长

Tāi Wěi Bù Zhǎng

Definition: Retarded growth of the fetus is characterized by slow growth of the fetus after four to five months of pregnancy. The gravida's abdominal size is significantly smaller than the normal size for the corresponding month of pregnancy. In Chinese medicine, it is called tai wei bu zhang.

Pathogenesis: Retarded growth of the fetus is usually caused by genetic defects, qi and blood deficiency, pi shen yang deficiency, heat toxins, etc.

Treatments Based on CM Diagnosis

Internal Treatments

(1) Qi Blood Deficiency

Zheng: After four to five months of pregnancy, the fetus is alive but the gravida's abdominal size is significantly smaller than the normal size for the corresponding month of pregnancy, the gravida's body is thin and weak, pale and yellow complexion, dizziness, shortness of breath, light red tongue, white thin tai, thin weak pulse.

Treatment method: Replenishing qi, nourishing the blood, and nurturing the fetus.

Formula: Ba zhen tang.

(2) Pi Shen Yang Deficiency

Zheng: After four to five months of pregnancy, the fetus is alive but the gravida's abdominal size is significantly smaller than the normal size for the corresponding month of pregnancy, anorexia, diarrhea, body cold, aversion to cold, cold limbs, light tongue, white tai, deep slow pulse.

Treatment method: Promoting the pi and warming the shen.

Formula: Wen tu yu lin tang.

(3) Blood Heat

Zheng: After four to five months of pregnancy, the fetus is alive but the gravida's abdominal size is significantly smaller than the normal size for the corresponding month of pregnancy, flushed complexion, red lips, vexation, dysphoria with feverish sensation on the chest, palms, and soles, dry mouth, thirst, red tongue, yellow tai, thin fast pulse.

Treatment method: Clearing heat and cooling the blood, nourishing yin and replenishing the blood.

Formula: Bao yin jian.

Hypogalactia

缺　乳

Quē Rǔ

Definition: Hypogalactia is characterized by little or no milk in the puerperium. In Chinese medicine, it is called que ru.

Pathogenesis: Hypogalactia is usually caused by weak qi and blood deficiency, gan qi stagnation, etc.

Treatments Based on CM Diagnosis

Internal Treatments

(1)　Qi Blood Deficiency

Zheng: Little or no milk in the puerperium, milk is thin if any, breasts are soft without distending sensation, pale complexion, listlessness, anorexia, light red tongue, white thin tai, weak thin pulse.

Treatment method: Replenishing qi, nourishing the blood, and promoting lactation.

Formula: Tong ru dan.

(2) Gan Qi Stagnancy

Zheng: Little or no milk in the puerperium, chest and hypochondriac distension, depression, low grade fever, anorexia, red tongue, thin yellow tai, stringy thin fast pulse.

Treatment method: Soothing the gan and resolving stagnation, opening channels and promoting lactation.

Formula: Xia ru yong quan san.

5. Surgery

Furunculosis

疖

Jiē

Definition: Furunculosis is characterized by acute suppurative cutaneous infection with redness, hotness, swelling, pain, shallow roots, and a range limited to about 3 cm. It can easily become pyogenic, diabrotic, and concentrated. It can be divided into you tou jie, wu tou jie, lou gu jie, and jie bing. In Chinese medicine, it is referred to as jie.

Pathogenesis: Furunculosis is usually caused by shi heat, feng, sweat obstruction, inappropriate hygiene, general asthenia, inappropriate or delayed treatments, etc.

Treatments Based on CM Diagnosis

Internal Treatments

(1) Heat Toxins

Zheng: A couple to multiple jie, distributed all over the body or concentrated in one area, chronic process, fever, thirst, yellow urine, constipation, red tongue, yellow tai, fast pulse.

Treatment method: Clearing heat and detoxifying.

Formula: Wu wei xiao du yin.

(2) Summer Heat

Zheng: Occurs in the summer to early fall, appears on the face and head, several to several dozens, red color, pain, swelling, shallow root, localized, round shape, becomes purulent in three to five days, exudes yellow pus, scabs in two to three days, may have yellow and white heads, accompanied by fever, headache, bitter mouth, dry throat, constipation, yellow urine, red tongue, yellow greasy tai, fast slippery pulse.

Treatment method: Clearing summer heat, resolving shi, and detoxifying.

Formula: Qing shu tang.

(3) Yin Deficiency

Zheng: Chronic process, occurs on and off, distributed around the body, large size, easily becomes you tou ju, thirst, dry lips, red tongue, thin tai, thin fast pulse.

Treatment method: Nourishing yin, clearing heat, and detoxifying.

Formula: Fang feng tong sheng san.

(4) Pi Wei Deficiency

Zheng: Distributed all over the body, slow diabrosis, slow healing, dilute pus, yellow complexion, fatigue, listlessness, anorexia, diarrhea, light red tongue, teeth prints, thin tai, soft pulse.

Treatment method: Promoting the pi and soothing the wei, clearing shi heat.

Formula: Fang feng tong sheng san.

External Treatments

(1)   Initial stage: Jin huang san, yu lu san, qian chui gao, or huang lian gao, etc.
(2)   Purulent stage: Incision and drainage.
(3)   Diabrotic stage: Jiu yi dan, tai yi gao.
(4)   Eczema: Qing dai san.

Facial Boil

颜 面 部 疔 疮

Yán Miàn Bù Dīng Chuāng

Definition: Facial boil is characterized by a small, hard, deep-rooted, nail-like furuncle on the face. Its progress is rapidly accompanied by fever, thirst, etc. In Chinese medicine, it is referred to as yan mian bu ding chuang.

Pathogenesis: Facial boil is usually caused by internal or external heat and huo toxins, which accumulate in the skin and muscles and block the qi movement and blood circulation.

The disease has the following stages:

(1) Initial stage: Rice-like purulent head on the face, itchy or numb, gradually becomes red, swollen, hot, and painful. It is 3 to 6 cm in size, has a deep root, and is hard and nail-like.

(2) Intermediate stage: After five to seven days, swelling increases, there is infiltration, pain increases, the purulent head ulcerates. Other symptoms include fever, aversion to cold, thirst, constipation, yellow urine, red tongue, yellow tai, stringy pulse.

(3) Final stage: After seven to ten days, it exudes pus, swelling is localized, the purulent core exudes pus, the furuncle root becomes soft, swelling reduces, fever decreases, and recovery occurs in ten to fourteen days. In some situations, if pressed or treated inappropriately, there may be septicemia, multiple abscess, or pyogenic infection of the bone.

Treatments Based on CM Diagnosis

Internal Treatments

(1) Heat Toxins

Zheng: Affected area is red and swollen, root concentrated, fever, headache, red tongue, yellow tai, fast pulse.

Treatment method: Clearing heat and detoxifying.

Formula: Wu wei xiao du yin and huang lian jie du tang.

(2) Huo Toxin Hyperactivity

Zheng: Affected area is flat, with diffuse swelling, and is dark purple, hot, and painful, high fever, headache, thirst, nausea, yellow urine, constipation, deep red tongue, yellow greasy tai, strong fast pulse.

Treatment method: Cooling the blood, clearing heat, and detoxifying.

Formula: Xi jiao di huang tang, huang lian jie du tang, and wu wei xiao du yin.

External Treatments

(1) Initial stage: Yu lu san, jin huang san, qian chui gao.
(2) Intermediate stage: Jiu yi dan, ba er dan, yu lu gao, qian chui gao, etc. Use incision and medical thread drainage if needed.
(3) Final stage: Sheng ji san, tai yi gao, hong you gao.

Hand and Foot Subcutaneous Abscess

手 足 部 疔 疮

Shǒu Zú Bù Dīng Chuāng

Definition: Hand and foot subcutaneous abscess is characterized by redness, swelling, pain, hotness, numbness, etc., on the hand or foot, which progresses to pyogenesis, aversion to cold, fever, headache, body ache, etc. If treated inappropriately, it may damage the bone and lead to dysfunction. In Chinese medicine, it is referred to as shou zu bu ding chuang.

Pathogenesis: Hand and food subcutaneous abscess is usually caused by shi huo toxins, blood stasis, and the patient may have a history of wounds and injuries.

Treatments Based on CM Diagnosis

Internal Treatments

(1) Huo Toxin Accumulation

Zheng: Localized redness, swelling, pain, aversion to cold, fever, red tongue, yellow tai, fast pulse.

Treatment method: Clearing heat and detoxifying.

Formula: Wu wei xiao du yin and huang lian jie du tang.

(2) Heat Hyperactivity and Flesh Decay

Zheng: Severe redness, swelling, and pain, pyogenesis. If the bone is not affected, swelling and pain will recede after diabrosis and pus exudes. If the bone is affected, swelling and pain remain after diabrosis, and pus exudes continuously. Red tongue, yellow tai, fast pulse.

Treatment method: Clearing heat, penetrating the pus, and driving out toxins.

Formula: Wu wei xiao du yin and huang lian jie du tang.

(3) Shi Heat Descending

Zheng: Planta is red, swollen, hot, and painful. Aversion to cold, fever, headache, anorexia, red tongue, yellow greasy tai, slippery fast pulse.

Treatment method: Clearing heat, detoxifying, and diuresis.

Formula: Wu shen tang and bi xie shen shi tang.

External Treatments

(1) Initial stage: Jin huang gao.
(2) Diabrosis stage: Incision and drainage, ba er dan or jiu yi dan medical thread, covered with jin huang gao or hong you gao.
(3) Healing stage: Sheng ji san, bai yu gao.
(4) Dead bone: Use qi san dan to clean the pus. When the dead bone is movable, remove it with medical forceps.

Acute Superficial Lymphangitis

红 丝 疔

Hóng Sī Dīng

Definition: Acute superficial lymphangitis is characterized by a red thread moving rapidly from the distal end to the proximal end of the extremities and body trunk. For the upper limbs, the red thread may stop at the elbow or armpit. For the lower limbs, it may stop at the popliteal fossa or groin. The condition is serious if the red thread is thick and moves towards the trunk. If accompanied by high fever, fainting, chest pain, hemoptysis, etc., septicemia is indicated. In Chinese medicine, it is referred to as hong si ding.

Pathogenesis: Acute superficial lymphangitis is usually caused by internal huo toxins together with furuncles or skin lesions on the extremities.

Treatments Based on CM Diagnosis

Internal Treatments

(1) Huo Toxins in Channels

Zheng: Thin red thread, mild whole body signs and symptoms, red tongue, thin yellow tai, soft fast pulse.

Treatment method: Clearing heat and detoxifying.

Formula: Wu wei xiao du yin.

(2) Huo Toxins in the Ying

Zheng: Red thread is thick and bulges out, red thread moves rapidly, chills, high fever, vexation, headache, thirst, deep red tongue, yellow greasy tai, strong fast pulse.

Treatment method: Cooling the blood and clearing the ying, detoxifying and dispersing toxins.

Formula: Xi jiao di huang tang, huang lian jie du tang, and wu wei xiao du yin.

External Treatments

(1) Thin red thread: Clean the skin with disinfection procedures. Cut and break the red thread with a knife and needles every inch. Squeeze the opening with the thumb and index fingers and let a small amount of blood out. Place tai yi gao, hong ling dan, and huang lian gao at the proximal broken end of the red thread.
(2) Purulent stage: Incision and drainage.
(3) Diabrotic stage: Use ba er dan or jiu yi dan, drain with medical thread, apply hong you gao. If there are connections between several diabrosis areas, bandage the areas or cut and break the connections. After the pus clear, apply sheng ji san and bai yu gao.

Gas Gangrene

烂 疔

Làn Dīng

Definition: Gas gangrene is characterized by sudden onset of hot, dark red swelling and pain, after which the skin turns black or with white patches, decays rapidly, affecting a large area, and slightly sinks. Dilute pus exudes after diabrosis. It easily develops into zou huang. In Chinese medicine, gas gangrene is referred to as lan ding.

Pathogenesis: Gas gangrene is usually caused by wounds, touching shi mud or dirty objects, special toxins, and shi heat hyperactivity.

Treatments Based on CM Diagnosis

Internal Treatments

(1) Shi Huo Hyperactivity

Zheng: Initially the affected limb feels heavy and tight. Gradual distending pain, the area is red, swollen, and bright. A large area of the skin sinks upon pressing. Severe pain after one to two days, blisters, decay, high fever, red tongue, thin white or yellow tai, stringy fast pulse.

Treatment method: Clearing heat, detoxifying, and diuresis.

Formula: Huang lian jie du tang and san miao wan.

(2) Toxins in Ying Blood

Zheng: High fever, headache, dizziness, delirium, shortness of breath, vexation, regurgitation, vomiting, swelling, pain, wound area is bright with severe edema, then becomes dark purple, bloody vesicles, muscle decay, dilute pus, with gas bubbles coming out, foul smell, deep red tongue, thin yellow tai, strong slippery fast pulse.

Treatment method: Cooling the blood and detoxifying, clearing heat and diuresis.

Formula: Xi jiao di huang tang, huang lian jie du tang, and san miao wan.

External Treatments

(1) Surgery removing all affected tissues.
(2) Washing with hydrogen dioxide solution.
(3) Filled up with gauze soaked with hydrogen dioxide solution.
(4) Use sheng ji san and hong you gao.

Cutaneous Anthrax

疫 疔

Yì Dīng

Definition: Cutaneous anthrax is characterized by insect bite blisters which rapidly dry and navel-like necrosis, with whole body symptoms. It is contagious and may develop into zou huang. In Chinese medicine, cutaneous anthrax is referred to as yi ding.

Pathogenesis: Cutaneous anthrax is usually caused when workers in livestock husbandry, butchers, tanners, etc., are affected by special toxins, leading to qi blood stasis and toxin accumulation.

Treatments Based on CM Diagnosis

Internal Treatments

(1) Heat Toxins

Zheng: Red papulae, itchiness, no pain, slight fever, papulae become blisters the next day, slight yellow liquid, swelling, fever, red tongue, yellow tai, fast pulse.

Treatment method: Clearing heat and detoxifying.

Formula: Wu wei xiao du yin and huang lian jie du tang.

(2) Huo Toxin Hyperactivity

Zheng: After three to four days, blisters dry up and turn into dark red or black necrosis, with groups of small grey-green blisters, skin sinks like a navel, enlarged diffuse swelling, soft without root, enlarged lymph nodes, high fever, headache, bone pain, deep red tongue, yellow greasy tai, strong fast pulse.

Treatment method: Cooling blood, clearing heat, and detoxifying.

Formula: Xi jiao di huang tang, huang lian jie du tang, and wu wei xiao du yin.

External Treatments

(1) Initial stage: Yu lu gao and chan su he ji or sheng dan.
(2) Putrefactive stage: Chan su he ji or wu wu dan.
(3) End stage: Sheng ji san.

Skin Superficial Abscess

Yōng

Definition: Skin superficial abscess is characterized by acute purulent infection in tissues and organs, with localized redness, swelling, hotness, and pain accompanied by some whole body symptoms. The disease area is localized around 6 to 9 cm. In Chinese medicine, it is referred to as yong.

Pathogenesis: Skin superficial abscess is usually caused by six external climate conditions in excess, diet with excessive fat, internal shi heat toxins, external toxins, etc.

Treatments Based on CM Diagnosis

Internal Treatments

(1) Initial Stage

Zheng: Sudden onset of discomfort under the skin, area is smooth and soft without a head, forming nodules quickly, bright red, hot, and painful, gradually swelling and hardening, may be accompanied by aversion to cold, fever, headache, nausea, red tongue, yellow greasy tai, strong fast pulse.

Treatment method: Driving out feng and clearing heat, moving the blood and eliminating stasis.

Formula: Xian fang huo ming yin.

(2) Purulent Stage

Zheng: Swelling is localized, soft when pressed, progressing pain, continuous fever, deep red tongue, dry yellow tai, powerful fast pulse.

Treatment method: Regulating the ying, clearing heat, and expelling toxins.

Formula: Tou nong san.

(3) Diabrotic Stage

Zheng: Thick yellow-whitish pus exudes which may be blended with blood, swelling reduces, pain recedes, whole body symptoms reduce, area scabs and heals gradually.

Treatment method: Nourishing qi and the blood.

Formula: Ba zhen tang.

External Treatments

(1) Initial stage: Jin huang gao, yu lu gao, qian chui gao, tai yi gao, hong ling dan, yang du nei xiao san.
(2) Purulent stage: Incision and drainage.
(3) Diabrotic stage: Apply ba er dan or jiu yi dan, drain with medical thread. After pus is cleared, apply sheng ji san, tai yi gao, sheng ji yu hong gao. If the pus cannot be drained completely, use debridement.

Cellulitis of the Floor of the Mouth

锁　喉　痈

Suǒ Hóu Yōng

Definition: Cellulitis of the floor of the mouth is characterized by acute onset of swelling around the prominentia laryngea, which is hot, painful, and rapidly progresses. It may affect the cheek and chest. Other symptoms are fever, thirst, headache, tight neck, constipation, shortness of breath, convulsion, etc. In Chinese medicine, cellulitis of the floor of the mouth is referred to as suo hou yong.

Pathogenesis: Cellulitis of the floor of the mouth is usually caused by feng heat toxins, measles, smallpox, chickenpox, deficiency conditions, etc.

Treatments Based on CM Diagnosis

Internal Treatments

(1) Tan Heat Accumulation

Zheng: Redness, diffuse swelling around the throat, hardness, high fever, thirst, headache, tight neck, constipation, yellow urine, deep red tongue, yellow greasy tai, stringy slippery fast or strong pulse.

Treatment method: Dispersing feng and clearing heat, dissolving tan and detoxifying.

Formula: Pu ji xiao du yin.

(2) Excessive Heat and Flesh Decaying

Zheng: Swelling is localized, soft upon pressure, thick yellow pus, heat recedes and swelling reduces, red tongue, yellow tai, fast pulse.

Treatment method: Clearing heat and dissolving phlegm, soothing the ying and driving out toxins.

Formula: Pu ji xiao du yin.

(3) Wei Yin Deficiency

Zheng: After diabrosis, pus is dilute, empty shell around the affected area, or pus exudes from the throat, heals slowly, anorexia, dry mouth, red tongue, little tai, thin pulse.

Treatment method: Clearing heat and nourishing wei yin.

Formula: Yi wei tang.

External Treatments

(1) Initial stage: Yu lu san, shuang bai san blended with jin yin hua lu.
(2) Pyogenesis stage: Incision and drainage with jiu yi dan medical thread, covered with jin huang gao or hong you gao.
(3) End stage: Sheng ji san, bai yu gao.

Buttock Cellulitis

臀 痈

Tún Yōng

Definition: Buttock cellulitis is characterized by swelling and pain around the buttocks, affecting walking, may be accompanied by other signs and symptoms, etc. In Chinese medicine, buttock cellulitis is referred to as tun yong.

Pathogenesis: Buttock cellulitis is usually caused by shi heat huo toxins, boils, furuncles, injection infection, etc.

Treatments Based on CM Diagnosis

Internal Treatments

(1) Shi Huo Accumulation

Zheng: Redness, swelling, and pain around the buttocks, most prominent in the center. Difficulty walking, aversion to cold, fever, headache, achy joints, anorexia, red tongue, yellow greasy tai, fast pulse.

Treatment method: Clearing heat and detoxifying, soothing the ying and dissolving shi.

Formula: Huang lian jie du tang and xian fang huo ming yin.

(2) Shi Tan Blockage

Zheng: Diffuse swelling, no redness, hard nodules, progresses slowly, no other symptoms, light red tongue, thin white greasy tai, moderate pulse.

Treatment method: Soothing the ying and moving the blood, diuresis and dissolving phlegm.

Formula: Xian fang huo ming yin.

(3) Qi Blood Deficiency

Zheng: After diabrosis, large pieces of decayed tissues shed, affected area is deep and large, forming an empty cavity, heals slowly, pale and yellow complexion, fatigue, listlessness, anorexia, light red tongue, thin white tai, thin pulse.

Treatment method: Regulating and nourishing qi blood.

Formula: Ba zhen tang.

External Treatments

(1) Initial stage: Yu lu gao or jin huang gao.
(2) Pyogenesis stage: Incision and drainage, covered with ba er dan, hong you gao.
(3) End stage: Sheng ji san, bai yu gao.

Pyogenic Infection of the Dorsum of the Hand

手 发 背

Shǒu Fā Bèi

Definition: Pyogenic infection of the dorsum of the hand is characterized by the entire dorsum of the hand experiencing diffuse swelling, hotness, redness, pain, no swelling at the palm. It may affect the tendon and bone. In Chinese medicine, pyogenic infection of the dorsum of the hand is referred to as shou fa bei.

Pathogenesis: Pyogenic infection of the dorsum of the hand is usually caused by feng huo shi heat or external infections.

Treatments Based on CM Diagnosis

Internal Treatments

(1) Shi Heat Blockage

Zheng: Dorsum of the hand experiences redness, swelling, heat, pain, pyogenesis, ulceration. Aversion to cold, fever, red tongue, yellow tai, fast pulse.

Treatment method: Clearing heat and detoxifying, soothing the ying and dissolving shi.

Formula: Wu wei xiao du yin and xian fang huo ming yin.

(2) Qi Blood Deficiency

Zheng: Chronic diffuse swelling of the dorsum of the hand, dilute pus, fatigue, light tongue, thin tai, thin pulse.

187

Treatment method: Regulating and nourishing qi and the blood.

Formula: Ba zhen tang.

External Treatments

(1) Initial stage: Jin huang gao or yu lu gao.
(2) Pyogenesis: Incision and drainage with ba er dan medical thread, cover with hong you gao.
(3) End stage: Sheng ji san, bai yu gao.

Pyogenic Infection of the Dorsum of the Foot

足 发 背

Zú Fā Bèi

Definition: Pyogenic infection of the dorsum of the foot is characterized by swelling, hotness, redness, pain of the dorsum of the foot. The sole is not affected. In Chinese medicine, pyogenic infection of the dorsum of the foot is referred to as zu fa bei.

Pathogenesis: Pyogenic infection of the dorsum of the foot is usually caused by shi heat, wounds, toxins, blood stasis, qi stagnation, etc.

Treatments Based on CM Diagnosis

Internal Treatment

Shi Heat Descending

Zheng: Dorsum of the foot experiences redness, swelling, hotness, pain, pyogenesis. Chills, fever, anorexia, nausea. After diabrosis, dilute pus exudes which may contain blood. Ulceration, red tongue, thin yellow greasy tai, slippery fast pulse.

Treatment method: Clearing heat and detoxifying, soothing the ying and diuresis.

Formula: Wu shen tang and bi xie shen shi tang.

External Treatments

(1) Initial stage: Jin huang gao or yu lu gao.
(2) Pyogenesis: Incision and drainage with ba er dan medical thread, cover with hong you gao.
(3) End stage: Sheng ji san, bai yu gao.

Carbuncle

有 头 疽

Yǒu Tóu Jū

Definition: A carbuncle is characterized by an initial rice-like purulent head on the skin, hot sensation, redness, swelling, pain, progressing to deeper layers and surrounding areas. After diabrosis, it looks like a lotus seedpod or honeycomb. It may occur at the neck, back, chest, abdomen, etc. In Chinese medicine, carbuncle is referred to as you tou ju.

Based on signs and symptoms, a carbuncle goes through four stages:

(1) Formation
(2) Pyogenesis
(3) Discharging
(4) Regeneration

Pathogenesis: Carbuncles are usually caused by the accumulation of feng heat, shi heat, huo toxins, zang fu toxins, a weak constitution, etc.

Treatments Based on CM Diagnosis

Internal Treatments

(1) Huo Toxin Accumulation

Zheng: Skin is red, swollen, protruded, hot, painful. It is limited to the local area. Pus is thick and yellow. Progresses rapidly. Accompanied by fever, thirst, yellow urine, deep red tongue, yellow tai, fast powerful pulse.

191

Treatment method: Clearing heat and purging huo, soothing the ying and driving out toxins.

Formula: Huang lian jie du tang and xian fang huo ming yin.

(2) Shi Heat Stagnation

Zheng: Localized skin redness, swelling, hot sensation, pain. Yellow pus, low fever in the morning and high fever in the evening, chest distress, nausea, red tongue, white or yellow greasy tai, soft fast pulse.

Treatment method: Clearing heat and resolving shi, soothing the ying and driving out toxins.

Formula: Xian fang huo ming yin.

(3) Yin Deficiency and Huo Flaming Up

Zheng: Slight swelling spreads, purple color, pain, progresses slowly, a little pus which may contain blood, fever, vexation, thirst, excessive drinking, constipation, yellow urine, red tongue, yellow dry tai, thin stringy pulse.

Treatment method: Nourishing yin and supplementing fluids, clearing heat and driving out toxins.

Formula: Zhu ye huang qi tang.

(4) Qi Deficiency and Toxin Stagnation

Zheng: Slight swelling spreads, dark grey color, heaviness, distension, numbness, progresses slowly, a little pus, easily forming cavity, chills, fever, frequent urination, thirst, excessive drinking, listlessness, pale complexion, light tongue, white or light yellow tai, fast weak pulse.

Treatment method: Reinforcing zheng and driving out toxins.

Formula: Tuo li xiao du san.

External Treatments

(1) Initial stage: For huo toxin and shi heat zheng, use jin huang gao. For yin deficiency and qi deficiency zheng, use chong he gao.
(2) Diabrotic stage: Add ba er dan or jiu yi dan. For dilute pus with green color, use qi san dan. Perform surgical removal if the pus cannot exude easily.
(3) After the pus is gone, use sheng ji gao, bai yu gao.

Acute Pyogenic Osteomyelitis

无 头 疽

Wú Tóu Jū

Definition: Acute pyogenic osteomyelitis is characterized by suppurative infections in the bones and joints with diffuse swelling, pain deep in the bones, unchanged skin color. Difficult to be reduced, slow diabrosis, slow convergence, may cause bone damage or joint deformation. In Chinese medicine, acute pyogenic osteomyelitis is referred to as wu tou ju.

Pathogenesis: Acute pyogenic osteomyelitis is usually caused by toxins from furuncles, boils, measles, scarlet fever, typhoid, etc, and gan shen deficiency, qi blood deficiency, etc.

Treatments Based on CM Diagnosis

Internal Treatments

(1) Shi Heat Stagnation

Zheng: Fever, chills, pain in the bone, inability to move, gradual swelling, unchanged skin color, hot to the touch, pain on pressure, pain on percussion, red tongue, yellow tai, fast pulse.

Treatment method: Clearing heat and resolving shi, removing stasis and clearing channels.

Formula: Xian fang huo ming yin and wu shen tang.

(2) Heat Toxin Hyperactivity

Zheng: One to two weeks after the disease starts, continuous high fever, swelling, severe pain, skin redness, hotness, pus is generated, red tongue, yellow greasy tai, strong fast pulse.

Treatment method: Clearing heat and resolving shi, soothing the ying and driving out toxins.

Formula: Huang lian jie du tang and xian fang huo ming yin.

(3) Suppurative Toxins Eroding the Bone

Zheng: After diabrosis, pus and fluid drip, may form sinuses, muscle atrophy, producing uneven dead bone, fatigue, listlessness, dizziness, palpitation, low fever, dark red tongue, thin tai, soft thin pulse.

Treatment method: Nourishing qi and the blood, clearing toxins.

Formula: Ba zhen tang.

External Treatments

(1) Initial stage: Use jin huang gao or yu lu gao. Fix the diseased limb with a splint.
(2) Purulent stage: Incision and drainage. Use qi san dan or ba er dan medical thread drainage. Covering with hong you gao or chong he gao.
(3) Post-purulent stage: Sheng ji san or bai yu gao.
(4) Sinus formation: Use qian jin san or wu wu dan medical thread. May use surgery debridement.

Deep Muscle Abscess

流 注

Liú Zhù

Definition: Deep muscle abscess is characterized by diffuse swelling, pain, normal skin color. It often occurs at the extremities and body trunk where there are dense muscles and tends to spread to multiple locations. In Chinese medicine, deep muscle abscess is referred to as liu zhu.

Pathogenesis: Deep muscle abscess is usually caused by summer shi toxins, furuncles, boils, wounds, postpartum infections, etc.

Treatments Based on CM Diagnosis

Internal Treatments

(1) Remaining Toxin Attack

Zheng: History of furuncles, carbuncles, boils, etc. Fever, thirst, or may be accompanied by coma, delirium, red tongue, yellow tai, full fast pulse.

Treatment method: Clearing heat and detoxifying, cooling the blood and opening channels.

Formula: Huang lian jie du tang and xi jiao di huang tang.

(2) Summer Shi Blockage

Zheng: Occurs between summer and autumn, chills, fever, head distension, chest distress, nausea, body and bone ache, may have miliaria alba, light red tongue, white greasy tai, slippery fast pulse.

195

Treatment method: Detoxifying, clearing summer heat, and resolving shi.

Formula: Qing shu tang.

(3) Blood Stasis

Zheng: History of over-exertion, wounds, or delivery. Diffuse swelling, skin is a mild red or purple, clots after diabrosis, light red tongue, thin white or yellow greasy tai, uneven or fast pulse.

Treatment method: Soothing the ying and moving the blood, removing stasis and opening channels.

Formula: Huo xue san yu tang.

External Treatments

(1) At the stage of swelling without bumps, use yu lu gao and jin huang gao.
(2) At the stage of swelling with bumps, use tai yi gao and hong ling dan.
(3) At the stage after pus is formed, incision and drainage of the pus by means of ba er dan medical thread. When the pus has cleared, use sheng ji san, cover with hong you gao.

Mumps

发 颐

Fā Yí

Definition: Mumps is characterized by swelling and pain in the parotid glands, accompanied by difficulty opening the mouth, high fever, dry mouth and thirst, anorexia, constipation, etc. In Chinese medicine, mumps is referred to as fa yi.

Pathogenesis: Mumps is usually caused by exogenous febrile disease and accumulation of heat toxins.

Treatments Based on CM Diagnosis

Internal Treatments

(1) Initial Stage

Zheng: Slight pain between the cheek and chin, tension, swelling, slight difficulty opening the mouth, thick exudates from the opening end of the parotid glands on the cheek mucosa, red tongue, slightly yellow tai, floating fast pulse.

Treatment method: Clearing heat and detoxifying.

Formula: Pu ji xiao du yin.

(2) Purulent Stage

Zheng: Pain between the cheek and chin increases, jumping pain, pain becomes severe with pressing, red skin, swelling increases, surface has a feeling of wave-like motion when pressing upon cheek mucosa has purulent exudates, red tongue, yellow tai, stringy fast pulse.

Treatment method: Expelling toxins and draining pus.

Formula: Pu ji xiao du yin, removing niu bang zi and zhi jiang can, and adding zao jiao ci and pangolin.

(3) Coma State

Zheng: Delayed or inappropriate treatments may lead to high fever and unconsciousness.

Treatment method: Cooling the ying and detoxifying, resolving tan and eliminating heat, nourishing yin and producing jin.

Formula: Qing ying tang.

External Treatments

(1) Initial stage: Jin huang gao or yu lu gao.
(2) Purulent stage: Incision and drainage.
(3) Diabrotic stage: Drain with ba er dan medical thread first, then apply jin huang gao. After pus is removed, apply sheng ji san and hong you gao. If mouth mucosa has purulent exudates, rinse the mouth with isotonic saline first, then apply qing chui kou san, four to five times a day.

Acute Reticular Lymphangitis

丹　毒

Dān Dú

Definition: Acute reticular lymphangitis is characterized by sudden onset of reddish skin on the limbs, head, face, as well as aversion to cold, fever, headache, bone pain, etc. In Chinese medicine, acute reticular lymphangitis is referred to as dan du.

Pathogenesis: Acute reticular lymphangitis is usually caused by blood heat, huo toxins, broken skin, wounds, etc.

Treatments Based on CM Diagnosis

Internal Treatments

(1)　Feng Heat Toxin Accumulation

Zheng: Head and facial skin is reddish, hot, swollen, painful, or with blisters. Aversion to cold, fever, eye swelling, difficulty opening eyes, red tongue, thin yellow tai, floating fast pulse.

Treatment method: Dispersing feng, clearing heat, and detoxifying.

Formula: Pu ji xiao du yin.

(2)　Shi Heat Toxin Accumulation

Zheng: Leg skin is reddish, swollen, hot, painful, or with blisters. Purpura, pyogenesis, may lead to necrosis, elephantiasis crus, fever, red tongue, yellow greasy tai, strong fast pulse.

Treatment method: Clearing heat, diuresis, and detoxifying.

Formula: Wu shen tang and bi xie shen shi tang.

(3) Fetal Huo Accumulation

Zheng: Occurs in neonatal babies, often affecting the buttock skin. Skin is red, swollen, hot, painful, or changing locations. High fever, vexation.

Treatment method: Cooling the blood, clearing heat, and detoxifying.

Formula: Xi jiao di huang tang and huang lian jie du tang.

External Treatments

(1) Jin huang san or yu lu san blended with jin yin hua lu.
(2) Necrosis: If there is pus, incision and drainage with jiu yi dan medical thread.
(3) Recurrent at low leg: Local sterilization first, then use qi xing zhen or san leng zhen to tap the skin.

Toxemia

走 黄

Zǒu Huáng

Definition: Toxemia is characterized by toxins spreading into the blood, organs, and system. In Chinese medicine, it is referred to as zou huang.

Pathogenesis: Toxemia is usually caused by inappropriate or delayed treatments, inappropriate management of furuncles, inappropriate diet, etc.

Treatments Based on CM Diagnosis

Internal Treatment

Toxins Entering the Blood

Zheng: Tip of furuncle is sunken and black, no pus, diffuse and soft swelling, spreads rapidly, dark red skin, chills, fever, headache, may be accompanied by vexation, or coma, convulsion, abdominal pain, bone pain, spasms, asthma, cough, blurred vision, cold extremities, deep red tongue, yellow rough tai, full fast pulse.

Treatment method: Cooling the blood, clearing heat, and detoxifying.

Formula: Xi jiao di huang tang, huang lian jie du tang, and wu wei xiao du yin.

External Treatments

(1) Apply ba er dan at the sunken black furuncle tip. Cover with jin huang gao. Apply jin huang san or yu lu san blended with cold water around the area.
(2) If pus forms, use jiu yi dan, ba er dan, yu lu gao, qian chui gao, etc. Use incision and medical thread drainage if needed.
(3) If pus has cleared, use sheng ji san, tai yi gao, hong you gao.

Septicemia

内 陷

Nèi Xiàn

Definition: Septicemia is characterized by toxins of the skin and external diseases spreading into the blood, organs, and system. In Chinese medicine, it is referred to as nei xian.

Pathogenesis: Septicemia is usually caused by zheng qi deficiency, heat toxins flaring up, delayed or inappropriate treatments, etc.

Treatments Based on CM Diagnosis

Internal Treatments

(1) Heat Toxin Dominance

Zheng: Carbuncle stages 1 to 2, flat tip, diffuse root, purple and stagnant, dry, no pus, hot, pain, fever, thirst, vexation, coma, delirium, hypochondriac pain, constipation, yellow urine, deep red tongue, yellow greasy or rough tai, full fast or stringy pulse.

Treatment method: Cooling the blood, clearing heat, and detoxifying.

Formula: Qing ying tang and huang lian jie du tang, an gong niu huang wan, and zi xue dan.

(2) Zheng Deficiency and Xie Dominance

Zheng: Carbuncle stages 2 to 3, little pus which cannot be exuded, dark color, swelling, pain, fever, chills, fatigue, anorexia, spontaneous perspiration, hypochondriac pain, coma, delirium, shortness of breath, light red tongue, yellow greasy tai, feeble fast pulse. Or cold extremities, diarrhea, frequent urination, normal temperature, light red tongue, dark greasy tai, deep thin pulse.

Treatment method: Nourishing qi and the blood, driving out toxins, clearing the xin and soothing the shen.

Formula: Tuo li xiao du san and an gong niu huang wan.

(3) Pi Shen Yang Deficiency

Zheng: Carbuncle stage 4, swelling reduces, pus exudes, pus is dark and diluted, no growth of new muscles, white and light wound, numbness, persistent deficient heat, listlessness, anorexia, abdominal pain, diarrhea, cold extremities, spontaneous perspiration, may be accompanied by shortness of breath, or coma, syncope, light tongue, thin white or little tai, deep thin or feeble big weak pulse.

Treatment method: Warming and nourishing the pi and shen.

Formula: Fu zi li zhong tang.

(4) Wei Yin Deficiency

Zheng: Carbuncle stage 4, swelling reduces, pus exudes, pus is dark and diluted, no growth of new muscles, white and light wound, numbness, persistent deficient heat, listlessness, anorexia, abdominal pain, mouth and tongue ulceration, dry mouth, deep red tongue, as clear as mirror tai, thin fast pulse.

Treatment method: Producing jin and nourishing the wei.

Formula: Yi wei tang.

External Treatments

(1) Initial stage: For huo toxin and shi heat zheng, use jin huang gao. For yin deficiency and qi deficiency zheng, use chong he gao.
(2) Diabrotic stage: Add ba er dan or jiu yi dan. For dilute pus with green color, use qi san dan. Perform surgical removal if the pus cannot exude easily.
(3) After the pus is gone, use sheng ji gao and bai yu gao.

Lymphoid Tuberculosis

瘰 疬

Luǒ Lì

Definition: Lymphoid tuberculosis is a chronic process characterized by a series of small nodules in the neck or behind the ears, with no pain and no redness. The nodules may exude clear pus after diabrosis, accompanied by rotting tissues, etc. In Chinese medicine, lymphoid tuberculosis is referred to as luo li.

Pathogenesis: Lymphoid tuberculosis is usually caused by gan qi stagnation, pi transport dysfunction, tan and shi accumulation.

Treatments Based on CM Diagnosis

Internal Treatments

(1) Qi Stagnation and Tan Accumulation

Zheng: In the initial stage, nodules are firm, with no obvious bodily symptoms. Light red tongue, yellow greasy tai, stringy slippery pulse.

Treatment method: Soothing the gan and regulating qi, resolving tan and dispersing nodules.

Formula: Xiao yao san and er chen tang.

(2) Yin Deficiency and Huo Flaming Up

Zheng: Nodules enlarge progressively and are attached to the skin, dark red skin, tidal fever in the afternoon, night sweats, red tongue, little tai, thin fast pulse.

Treatment method: Nourishing yin and descending huo.

Formula: Liu wei di huang wan and qing gu san.

(3) Qi and Blood Deficiency

Zheng: Diseased area exudes clear pus with rotting tissues, weight loss, listlessness, pale complexion, light tongue, thin tai, thin pulse.

Treatment method: Nourishing qi and replenishing the blood.

Formula: Xiang bei yang ying tang.

External Treatments

(1) Initial stage: Chong he gao.
(2) Middle stage: Chong he gao or qian chui gao.
(3) Diabrotic stage: Use wu wu dan or qi san dan, then use ba er dan medical drainage thread.
(4) End stage: Sheng ji san and bai yu gao.

Bone Tuberculosis
流　痰
Liú Tán

Definition: Bone tuberculosis is characterized by vague pain in the bone or joints, gradual joint dysfunction, normal skin color, slow pyogenesis, clear pus with cotton-like material, ulceration which has difficulty healing, easily causing sinus, may damage the bone and lead to disability, or may even be fatal. In Chinese medicine, bone tuberculosis is referred to as liu tan.

Pathogenesis: Bone tuberculosis is usually caused by shen deficiency, wounds, over-exertion, feng cold and shi attack.

Treatments Based on CM Diagnosis

Internal Treatments

(1) Yang Deficiency and Tan Accumulation

Zheng: Initially no redness, no hotness, no swelling, only slight vague pain in the bone or joints. Gradual joint dysfunction, pain increases, light tongue, thin tai, weak thin pulse.

Treatment method: Nourishing the shen and warming channels, driving out cold and resolving phlegm.

Formula: Yang he tang.

(2) Yin Deficiency and Internal Heat

Zheng: Gradual swelling, light red skin, pus forms, tidal fever in the afternoon, cheek redness, night sweats, dry mouth and throat, poor appetite, cough, mucus with blood, red tongue, little tai, thin fast pulse.

Treatment method: Nourishing yin, clearing heat, and driving out toxins.

Formula: Liu wei di huang wan, qing gu san, and tou nong san.

(3) Gan Shen Deficiency

Zheng: After diabrosis, clear pus exudes with cotton-like material, forming sinuses, muscle atrophy, deformation, or paralysis, waste retention or incontinence, weight loss, pale complexion, aversion to cold, palpitation, insomnia, spontaneous perspiration, night sweats, light red tongue, white tai, thin fast or empty pulse.

Treatment method: Replenishing the gan and shen.

Formula: Zuo gui wan and xiang bei yang ying tang.

External Treatments

(1) Initial stage: Hui yang yu long gao.
(2) Middle stage: Incision drainage.
(3) Late stage: After diabrosis, use wu wu dan medical thread. Then use sheng ji san.
(4) Sinus: Wu wu dan medial thread.

Acute Mastitis

乳 痈

Rǔ Yōng

Definition: Acute mastitis is characterized by breast nodules, redness, swelling, hotness, pain, fever, tight chest, headache, fast temper, anorexia, constipation, or may be accompanied by pyogenesis, ulceration, etc. If treated inappropriately, it may result in fistulae and pyosepticemia, etc. In Chinese medicine, acute mastitis is referred to as ru yong.

Pathogenesis: Acute mastitis is usually caused by milk accumulation, emotional distress, inappropriate diet, external toxins, etc.

Treatments Based on CM Diagnosis

Internal Treatments

(1) Qi Stagnation and Heat Accumulation

Zheng: Chunks accumulate in breast milk, skin color is normal or a mild red, swelling and pain, aversion to cold, fever, headache, body ache, thirst, constipation, light red tongue, thin tai, fast pulse.

Treatment method: Soothing the gan and clearing the wei, moving milk and reducing swelling.

Formula: Gua lou niu bang tang.

(2) Heat Toxin Hyperactivity

Zheng: High fever, breast is swollen, painful, red, and hot, soft nodules, or incision drainage is not smooth, inflammation does not reduce and spreads to other collaterals, red tongue, yellow greasy tai, powerful fast pulse.

Treatment method: Clearing heat and detoxifying, driving inside xie out and removing pus.

Formula: Tou nong san.

(3) Zheng Deficiency and Lingering Toxins

Zheng: After diabrosis, swelling and pain reduce, but pus fluid exudes continuously, pus is clear, heals slowly, may forming fistulae, fatigue, pale complexion, low fever, poor appetite, light tongue, thin tai, weak pulse.

Treatment method: Nourishing qi, soothing the ying, and driving out toxins.

Formula: Tuo li xiao du san.

External Treatments

(1) Initial stage: Hot compress, massage, jin huang gao, yu lu gao, etc.
(2) Pyogenesis stage: Incision drainage.
(3) Diabrosis stage: After incision drainage, use ba er dan or jiu yi dan medical thread, cover with jin huang gao.
(4) End stage: Sheng ji san, cover with hong you gao or sheng ji yu hong gao.

Mammary Phlegmon

乳发

Rǔ Fā

Definition: Mammary phlegmon is characterized by red breast skin, diffuse swelling, severe pain, sunken sweat pores, rapid ulceration and gangrene, or heat toxin internal attack, etc. In Chinese medicine, mammary phlegmon is referred to as ru fa.

Pathogenesis: Mammary phlegmon is usually caused by loss of jing and blood, shi heat huo toxins, seasonal pestilences, gan qi stagnation, inappropriate diet, etc.

Treatments Based on CM Diagnosis

Internal Treatments

(1) Heat Toxin Accumulation

Zheng: Red breast skin, diffuse swelling, severe pain, sunken sweat pores, fever, headache, constipation, yellow urine, red tongue, yellow tai, slippery fast pulse.

Treatment method: Clearing heat and detoxifying.

Formula: Huang lian jie du tang.

(2) Huo Toxin Hyperactivity

Zheng: After a few days, breast skin is shi and ulcerated, becoming black and gangrenous, increased pain, high fever, thirst, deep red tongue, yellow dry tai, fast pulse.

Treatment method: Purging huo and detoxifying.

Formula: Long dan xie gan tang and huang lian jie du tang.

(3) Zheng Deficiency and Lingering Xie

Zheng: After appropriate treatments, fever is gone, swelling reduces, some new tissue grows, color is not bright, heals slowly, fatigue, listlessness, pale complexion, light tongue, thin tai, soft thin pulse.

Treatment method: Nourishing qi, soothing the ying, and driving out toxins.

Formula: Tuo li xiao du san.

External Treatments

(1) Initial stage: Yu lu gao.
(2) Pyogenesis stage: Incision drainage, qi san dan or wu wu dan medical thread, cover with yu lu gao.
(3) Diabrosis stage: Qi san dan and yu lu gao first. Then use sheng ji san and hong you gao.

Tuberculosis of the Breast

乳 癆

Rǔ Láo

Definition: Tuberculosis of the breast is characterized by breast nodules at the beginning, gradual pyogenesis, ulceration exuding dilute pus, and accompanied by some bodily signs and symptoms. In Chinese medicine, tuberculosis of the breast is referred to as ru lao.

Pathogenesis: Tuberculosis of the breast is usually caused by yin, qi, and blood deficiency, and attacks by external toxins, or is secondary to other kinds of tuberculosis, etc.

Treatments Based on CM Diagnosis

Internal Treatments

(1) Qi Stagnation and Tan Accumulation

Zheng: In the initial stage, breast nodules, no redness, no hotness, no pain, stress, tightness and distress in the chest, hypochondriac distension, light tongue, thin greasy tai, stringy slippery pulse.

Treatment method: Soothing the gan and resolving stagnation, dissolving tan and dispersing nodules.

Formula: Kai yu san and xiao li wan.

(2) Yin Deficiency and Tan Hotness

Zheng: After pyogenesis or diabrosis, skin is dark red, nodule becomes soft, exudes dilute pus with old cotton-like material, hectic fever, night sweats, fatigue, listlessness, cheek redness, emaciation, anorexia, red tongue, yellow tai, thin fast pulse.

Treatment method: Nourishing yin, clearing heat, and dissolving phlegm.

Formula: Liu wei di huang wan and qing gu san.

External Treatments

(1) Initial stage: Yang he jie ning gao and gui she san or hei tui xiao.
(2) Pyogenesis stage: Incision and drainage.
(3) Diabrosis stage: Hong you gao and wu wu dan. Then use sheng ji san and hong you gao.
(4) Fistula: Bai jiang dan or hong sheng dan medical thread. Then use sheng ji san.

Fibroadenoma of the Breast

乳 核

Rǔ Hé

Definition: Fibroadenoma of the breast is characterized by egg-shaped nodules inside the breast, with clear borders, smooth surfaces, and are movable upon pressing. In Chinese medicine, fibroadenoma of the breast is referred to as ru he.

Pathogenesis: Fibroadenoma of the breast is usually caused by emotional stress, gan qi stagnation, anxiety, chong and ren channel disorder, etc.

Treatments Based on CM Diagnosis

Internal Treatments

(1) Gan Qi Stagnation

Zheng: Small nodules which grow slowly and are not red, not hot, not painful, and movable upon pressing. Discomfort in the breast, chest distress, sighing, light red tongue, thin white tai, stringy pulse.

Treatment method: Soothing the gan and resolving stagnation.

Formula: Xiao yao san.

(2) Blood Stasis amd Tan Accumulation

Zheng: Large nodules which are firm and hard. Heaviness, discomfort, tightness and pain in the chest, vexation, fast temper, irregular menstruation, dysmenorrhea, dark red tongue, thin greasy tai, stringy thin pulse.

Treatment method: Soothing the gan and moving the blood, dissolving tan and dispersing nodules.

Formula: Xiao yao san and tao hong si wu tang.

Hyperplasia of the Mammary Glands

乳 癖

Rǔ Pǐ

Definition: Hyperplasia of the mammary glands is characterized by pain in one or both breasts and the presence of nodules. The nodules vary in size and shape, have unclear borders, are not very firm, are movable, and are associated with the menstrual cycle and emotional change. It may evolve to breast cancer. In Chinese medicine, hyperplasia of the mammary glands is referred to as ru pi.

Pathogenesis: Hyperplasia of the mammary glands is usually caused by emotional distress, gan qi stagnation, blood stasis, chong ren disharmony, etc.

Treatments Based on CM Diagnosis

Internal Treatments

(1) Gan Stagnation and Tan Accumulation

Zheng: Often seen in young and robust women, nodules fluctuate with emotions, chest distress, hypochondriac distension, anxiety, fast temper, insomnia, excessive dreaming, vexation, bitter taste, red tongue, thin yellow tai, stringy slippery pulse.

Treatment method: Soothing the gan and clearing stagnation, dissolving tan and dispersing nodules.

Formula: Xiao yao lou bei san.

217

(2) Chong Ren Disharmony

Zheng: Often seen in middle-aged women, nodules get worse before periods and are relieved after periods, soreness in the waist, fatigue, listlessness, irregular menstruation, scanty period with light color, or amenorrhea, light tongue, white tai, deep thin pulse.

Treatment method: Regulate the chong ren.

Formula: Er xian tang and si wu tang.

Hypermastia

乳 疬

Rǔ Lì

Definition: Hypermastia is characterized by oval lumps at one or both areola of mamma, intermediate hardness, slight pressing pain. In Chinese medicine, hypermastia is referred to as ru li.

Pathogenesis: Hypermastia is usually caused by gan qi stagnation, phlegm, shen deficiency, etc.

Treatments Based on CM Diagnosis

Internal Treatments

(1) Gan Qi Stagnation

Zheng: Pain in the breast lumps which increases upon pressing, fast temper, chest and hypochondriac radiating pain, red tongue, white tai, stringy pulse.

Treatment method: Soothing the gan and dispersing lumps.

Formula: Xiao yao lou bei san.

(2) Shen Yang Deficiency

Zheng: Often seen in middle-aged and senior patients, pale complexion, soreness in the waist and legs, fatigue, light tongue, white tai, deep weak pulse.

Treatment method: Nourishing shen yang.

Formula: You gui wan.

(3) Shen Yin Deficiency

Zheng: Usually seen in middle-aged or senior patients, dizziness, dysphoria with feverish sensation in the chest, palms, and soles, insomnia, excessive dreaming, red tongue, little tai, stringy thin pulse.

Treatment method: Nourishing shen yin.

Formula: Zuo gui wan.

Fistula of the Breast

乳 漏

Rǔ Lòu

Definition: Fistula of the breast is characterized by a chronic fistula of the breast, with difficulty healing after diabrosis of opening sores, exuding pus which may be mixed with milk or bean-dregs-like exudates. In Chinese medicine, fistula of the breast is referred to as ru lou.

Pathogenesis: Fistula of the breast is usually caused by inappropriate treatments of acute mastitis, mammary phlegmon, tuberculosis of the breast, etc., genetic abnormality, toxins, etc.

Treatments Based on CM Diagnosis

Internal Treatments

(1) Yin Deficiency and Lingering Xie

Zheng: After diabrosis in tuberculosis of the breast, exudes clear pus continuously which is hard to heal, or exudes pus which is mixed with worn cotton-like material, fatigue, tidal fever, night sweats, red tongue, thin yellow tai, thin fast pulse.

Treatment method: Nourishing yin and clearing heat.

Formula: Liu wei di huang wan and qing gu san.

(2) Qi Blood Deficiency

Zheng: After diabrosis in acute mastitis and mammary phlegmon, fistula forms, sores are hard to heal, exudes pus, blood, or milk, granulation not fresh, pale complexion, fatigue, light tongue, thin tai, soft pulse.

Treatment method: Nourishing qi and supplementing the blood, expelling from within and driving out pus.

Formula: Shi quan da bu tang and tuo li xiao du san.

External Treatments

(1) Qi san dan or ba er dan medical thread. Cover with hong you gao.
(2) After the pus is drained, use sheng ji san and sheng ji yu hong gao.
(3) Surgery if the above methods are ineffective.

Intracanalicular Papilloma

乳衄

Rǔ Nù

Definition: Intracanalicular papilloma is characterized by nipple secretion of bloody fluid, or with a lump around the areola of mamma. It is a benign tumor, but may become malignant in some cases. In Chinese medicine, intracanalicular papilloma is referred to as ru nu.

Pathogenesis: Intracanalicular papilloma is usually caused by stress, depression, anxiety, anger, etc.

Treatments Based on CM Diagnosis

Internal Treatments

(1) Gan Stagnation and Huo Hyperactivity

Zheng: Nipple secretes red or dark red fluid, vexation, fast temper, tightness and distress in the chest, hypochondriac pain, insomnia, excessive dreaming, red tongue, thin yellow tai, stringy pulse.

Treatment method: Soothing the gan and resolving stagnation, cooling the blood and hemostasis.

Formula: Dan zhi xiao yao san.

(2) Pi and Blood Deficiency

Zheng: Nipple secretes light red or yellow fluid, pale complexion, fatigue, anorexia, dysphoria, insomnia, light tongue, white tai, thin weak pulse.

Treatment method: Promoting the pi, nourishing the blood, and hemostasis.

Formula: Gui pi tang.

External Treatment

Surgery is indicated if the internal treatment is ineffective.

Breast Cancer

乳 岩

Rǔ Yán

Definition: Breast cancer may not show any symptoms at the early stage. As it progresses, it is characterized by mild to severe pain, nodules, lumps, enlarged lymph nodes, discharge and overflow, changes in the skin, etc. In Chinese medicine, breast cancer is referred to as ru yan, etc.

Pathogenesis: Breast cancer is usually caused by emotional stress, external toxin attacks, diet, etc.

Treatments Based on CM Diagnosis

Internal Treatments

(1) Chong Ren Irregularity

Zheng: Lump in the breast which is hard, connected to neighboring tissues, with a non-smooth surface. Dysphoria with feverish sensation in the chest, palms, and soles, tidal fever in the afternoon, night sweats, dry mouth, soreness in the waist and knees, irregular menstruation, fissured tongue, little tai, thin fast weak pulse.

Treatment method: Nourishing yin and descending huo, softening hardness and detoxifying.

Formula: Zhi bo di huang tang.

(2) Gan Qi Stagnation

Zheng: Breast lump distending pain, radiating to the chest and hypochondria, depression, fast temper, vexation, irritation, bitter taste, dry throat, dizziness, light dark tongue, thin white or yellow tai, stringy slippery pulse.

Treatment method: Soothing the gan and regulating qi, dissolving tan and dispersing lumps.

Formula: Xiao yao san.

(3) Heat Toxin Stasis

Zheng: Breast lump grows quickly, pain, redness, swelling, or ulceration, foul-smelling exudates, constipation, fever, dark red tongue, thin yellow tai, stringy fast pulse.

Treatment method: Clearing heat and detoxifying, removing stasis and reducing swelling.

Formula: Tao hong si wu tang and wu wei xiao du yin.

(4) Qi Blood Deficiency

Zheng: Breast lump is connected to the chest wall and resists pressures, breast skin grows small nodules, dizziness, pale complexion, fatigue, shortness of breath, light swollen tongue, little tai, weak pulse.

Treatment method: Nourishing qi and supplementing the blood, detoxifying and dispersing lumps.

Formula: Bu zhong yi qi tang.

Goiter

气 瘿

Qì Yǐng

Definition: Goiter is characterized by diffuse swelling of the neck, which is soft with no pain. The swelling changes with emotions. In Chinese medicine, goiter is referred to as qi ying.

Pathogenesis: Goiter is usually caused by emotion distress, iodine deficiency in the diet, postpartum shen deficiency, etc.

Treatments Based on CM Diagnosis

Internal Treatments

(1) Gan Stagnation and Pi Deficiency

Zheng: Diffuse swelling around the neck, fatigue, fondness for sighing, shortness of breath, anorexia, emaciation, pale complexion, thin white tai, weak pulse.

Treatment method: Soothing the gan and resolving stagnation, promoting the pi and strengthening qi.

Formula: Si hai shu yu wan.

(2) Gan Stagnation and Shen Deficiency

Zheng: Neck nodules are soft, sluggish, fatigue, aversion to cold, slow movement, cold extremities, decreased libido, light tongue, deep thin pulse.

Treatment method: Soothing the gan and nourishing the shen, regulating the chong ren.

Formula: Si hai shu yu wan and you gui yin.

External Treatment

If the internal treatment is ineffective, may try surgery.

Thyroid Adenoma

肉　瘿

Ròu Yǐng

Definition: Thyroid adenoma is characterized by nodules on one or both sides of the laryngeal protuberance, which are soft, round, move up and down with swallowing, and progress slowly. In Chinese medicine, thyroid adenoma is referred to as rou ying.

Pathogenesis: Thyroid adenoma is usually caused by anxiety, depression, anger, etc.

Treatments Based on CM Diagnosis

Internal Treatments

(1) Qi Stagnation and Tan Accumulation

Zheng: Nodules on the sides of the laryngeal protuberance, no redness, no hotness, no pain, moving up and down with swallowing, respiration difficulty, swallowing difficulty, light tongue, thin greasy tai, stringy slippery pulse.

Treatment method: Regulating qi and resolving stagnation, dissolving tan and softening hardness.

Formula: Xiao yao san and hai zao yu hu tang.

(2) Qi Yin Deficiency

Zheng: Soft neck nodules, fast temper, aversion to heat, perspiring easily, bitter taste, palpitation, insomnia, excessive dreaming, shaking hands, increased appetite, emaciation, irregular menstruation, red tongue, thin tai, stringy pulse.

Treatment method: Nourishing qi and supplementing yin, softening hardness and dispersing nodules.

Formula: Sheng mai san and hai zao yu hu tang.

External Treatment

Use gui she san.

Thyroiditis

瘿 痈

Yǐng Yōng

Definition: Thyroiditis is characterized by acute onset of nodules around the laryngeal protuberance, swelling, hotness, pain, etc. In Chinese medicine, thyroiditis is referred to as ying yong.

Pathogenesis: Thyroiditis is usually caused by feng heat, feng huo, wei heat, tan heat, etc.

Treatments Based on CM Diagnosis

Internal Treatments

(1) Feng Heat and Tan Accumulation

Zheng: Nodule pain, aversion to cold, fever, headache, thirst, dry throat, red tongue, thin yellow tai, floating fast or slippery fast pulse.

Treatment method: Dispersing feng, clearing heat, and dissolving phlegm.

Formula: Niu bang jie ji tang.

(2) Qi Stagnation and Tan Accumulation

Zheng: Firm nodules, slight swelling, pressing pain radiating to the occiput, blockage sensation in the throat, increased phlegm, light red tongue, yellow greasy tai, stringy slippery pulse.

Treatment method: Clearing the gan and regulating qi, dissolving tan and dispersing nodules.

Formula: Chai hu qing gan tang.

External Treatments

(1) Initial stage: Jin huang san, si huang san, or shuang bo san.
(2) Pyogenic stage: Incision and drainage with ba er dan medical thread, cover with jin huang gao.
(3) End stage: Sheng ji san, hong you gao.

Thyroid Carcinoma

石 瘿

Shí Yǐng

Definition: Thyroid carcinoma is characterized by hard nodules around the laryngeal protuberance, which are immovable and uneven. It may accompany other systemic signs and symptoms. In Chinese medicine, thyroid carcinoma is referred to as shi ying.

Pathogenesis: Thyroid carcinoma is usually caused by emotional distress, qi stagnation, blood stasis, phlegm, thyroid adenoma, etc.

Treatments Based on CM Diagnosis

Internal Treatments

(1) Tan Stasis

Zheng: Neck nodules grow quickly, are hard like stones, uneven, and immovable. No obvious bodily symptoms. Dark red tongue, thin yellow tai, stringy pulse.

Treatment method: Resolving stagnation and dissolving phlegm, moving the blood and reducing hardness.

Formula: Hai zao yu hu tang.

(2) Stasis Heat Damaging Yin

Zheng: Advanced stage, nodules are ulcerated, exuding blood and fluid, or metastasized. Fatigue, leanness, hoarse voice, purple dark tongue with ecchymosis, little tai, deep uneven pulse.

233

Treatment method: Soothing the ying and nourishing yin.

Formula: Tong qiao huo xue tang and yang yin qing fei tang.

External Treatments

(1) Use yang he jie ning gao.
(2) For pain and hotness, use crushed raw phytolacca root.

Neurofibromatosis

气 瘤

Qì Liú

Definition: Neurofibromatosis is characterized by multiple nodules under the skin, which are soft, sink upon pressing, and rebound upon releasing. In Chinese medicine, neurofibromatosis is referred to as qi liu.

Pathogenesis: Neurofibromatosis is usually caused by over-exertion, anxiety, cold, etc.

Treatments Based on CM Diagnosis

Internal Treatments

(1) Fei Qi Irregularity

Zheng: Superficial nodules which are floating and white in color. Pale complexion, fatigue, shortness of breath, spontaneous perspiration, aversion to cold, excessive clear phlegm, light red tongue, thin white tai, weak pulse.

Treatment method: Dispersing the fei and regulating qi, enriching qi and arresting the qi in the surface.

Formula: Tong qi san jian wan and yu ping feng san.

(2) Pi Deficiency and Tan Accumulation

Zheng: Multiple nodules, deeper roots, soft, no pain on touching, relief with warmth. Heavy head, fatigue, no thirst, no taste in the mouth, abdominal distension, diarrhea, light tongue, thin greasy tai, soft pulse.

Treatment method: Promoting the pi and resolving stagnation, dissolving tan and dispersing nodules.

Formula: Shi quan liu qi yin.

External Treatments

(1) For protruded nodules with small roots, use a thread to ligate the roots of the nodules.
(2) Surgery is indicated if the above treatment is ineffective.

Hemangioma

血 瘤

Xuè Liú

Definition: Hemangioma is characterized by a tumor of the dilated, cross-linked vessels on the skin. The area is red or dark purple, soft, with a blurred border, and a spongy feeling to the touch. In Chinese medicine, hemangioma is referred to as xue liu.

Pathogenesis: Hemangioma is usually caused by xin huo, fetus huo, gan stagnation, etc.

Treatments Based on CM Diagnosis

Internal Treatments

(1) Xin Huo Hyperactivity

Zheng: Tumor bright red, hot sensation, vexation, sores on the mouth and tongue, flushing, thirst, scanty yellow urine, constipation, red tongue, thin yellow tai, fast powerful pulse.

Treatment method: Clearing the xin and purging huo, cooling the blood and dispersing stasis.

Formula: Qin lian er mu wan and xie xin tang.

(2) Shen Huo Stagnation

Zheng: Tumor existing at birth on the face and/or neck, hotness, dysphoria with feverish sensation in the chest, palms, and soles, tidal fever, night sweats, slow growth, yellow urine, constipation, red tongue, little tai, thin fast pulse.

Treatment method: Nourishing yin and descending huo, cooling the blood and dissolving stasis.

Formula: Liang xue di huang tang and liu wei di huang wan.

(3) Gan Huo Hyperactivity

Zheng: Tumor is nevus-like or formed by dilated, twisted, curved vessels, expandable upon pressing, distending pain with emotional distress or anger, chest and hypochondriac discomfort, dry throat, scanty yellow urine, constipation, red tongue, yellow dry tai, stringy fast or thin pulse.

Treatment method: Clearing the gan, cooling the blood, and removing stasis.

Formula: Liang xue di huang tang and dan zhi xiao yao san.

External Treatments

(1) For small tumor not on the head or joints, may use wu miao shui xian gao.

(2) Surgery is indicated if the above treatment is ineffective.

Varicosis

筋 瘤

Jīn Liú

Definition: Varicosis is characterized by lumps of twisted veins on the skin, often occurring in the lower limbs, appearing dark red, moistured, may be protruded, forming groups, and are like earthworms. In Chinese medicine, varicosis is referred to as jin liu.

Pathogenesis: Varicosis is usually caused by gan shen deficiency, long periods of standing, over-exertion, multiple pregnancies, feng cold, etc.

Treatments Based on CM Diagnosis

Internal Treatments

(1) Huo Hyperactivity Burning the Blood

Zheng: Twisted veins are hot, dysphoria with feverish sensation in the chest, palms, and soles, dry mouth, red tongue, yellow tai, thin fast pulse.

Treatment method: Clearing the gan and purging huo, nourishing the blood and soothing tendons.

Formula: Qing gan lu hui wan and huang lian e jiao tang.

(2) Exertion Damaging Qi

Zheng: Twisted veins get worse after long periods of standing or walking, descending and discomfort increase, appearing light dark color, no increase in temperature, shortness of breath, fatigue, abdominal distending and descending, soreness in the waist, swollen tongue, light tongue, thin white tai, thin soft weak pulse.

Treatment method: Enforcing the middle jiao and strengthening qi, moving the blood and soothing tendons.

Formula: Bu zhong yi qi tang and si wu tang.

(3) Cold Shi Accumulation

Zheng: Dark purple lump, fondness for warmth, swollen legs, cold extremities, no taste, lack of thirst, clear urine, dark tongue, white greasy tai, stringy thin pulse.

Treatment method: Warming the gan and driving out cold, moving the blood and opening channels.

Formula: Nuan gan jian and si ni san.

External Treatments

(1) Wrap the leg with elastic bandages.
(2) For complications, please use treatments for the complications.

Myofibroma

肉 瘤

Ròu Liú

Definition: Myofibroma is characterized by soft masses under the skin, swelling like buns, unchanged skin color, no tightness, etc. In Chinese medicine, myofibroma is referred to as rou liu.

Pathogenesis: Myofibroma is usually caused by anxiety, inappropriate diet, over-exertion, anger, etc.

Treatments Based on CM Diagnosis

Internal Treatments

(1) Pi Deficiency and Tan Shi

Zheng: Relatively large mass, soft, broad root, no pain on touching, fondness for warmth and pressure. Pale yellow complexion, fatigue, shortness of breath, light red tongue, thin white tai, relaxed weak pulse.

Treatment method: Promoting the pi and opening the middle jiao, drying shi and resolving phlegm.

Formula: Gui pi tang and er chen tang.

(2) Gan Stagnant and Tan Accumulation

Zheng: Small multiple masses, relatively hard, slight pain on pressing, depression, vexation, fast temper, chest distress, sighing, red tongue, thin yellow tai, stringy pulse.

Treatment method: Soothing the gan, moving qi, and resolving stagnation.

Formula: Shi quan liu qi yin.

External Treatments

Use yang he jie ning gao.

Steatoma

脂 瘤

Zhī Liú

Definition: Steatoma is characterized by a mass under the skin, which is ball-shaped, with a clear border, movable, slow-growing, etc. In Chinese medicine, steatoma is referred to as zhi liu.

Pathogenesis: Steatoma is usually caused by blockage of the sudoriferous glands, pi maltransportation, scratching, etc.

Treatments Based on CM Diagnosis

Internal Treatments

(1) Tan Qi Accumulation

Zheng: Black spot on the mass, throat blockage, chest distress, emotional stress, fast temper, light tongue, greasy tai, slippery pulse.

Treatment method: Regulating qi, dissolving phlegm, and dispersing the mass.

Formula: Er chen tang and si qi tang.

(2) Tan Shi Heat

Zheng: Mass is red, hot, painful, with throbbing pain. Fever, aversion to cold, headache, yellow urine, red tongue, thin yellow tai, fast pulse.

Treatment method: Clearing heat and diuresis, moving the blood and removing stasis.

Formula: Long dan xie gan tang and xian fang huo ming yin.

External Treatments

(1) Surgery if no toxins.
(2) With toxins, jin huang gao or yu lu gao.
(3) Pyogenic stage: Incision and drainage.

Osteoma

骨　瘤

Gǔ Liú

Definition: Osteoma is characterized by a localized hard nodule in the bone, which is uneven, immovable, closely attached to the bone. In Chinese medicine, osteoma is referred to as gu liu.

Pathogenesis: Osteoma is usually caused by genetic deficiency, phlegm, shi, toxins, wounds, shen yin deficiency, etc.

Treatments Based on CM Diagnosis

Internal Treatment

Shen Deficiency

Zheng: Localized hard nodule in the bone, which is uneven, immovable, closely attached to the bone. Pain, dysfunction of the affected bone.

Treatment method: Nourishing the shen and removing stasis.

Formula: Tiao yuan shen qi wan.

External Treatments

(1) Hei tui xiao and yang he jie ning gao.
(2) Surgery is indicated if the above treatment is ineffective.

6. Anorectal Diseases

Internal Hemorrhoid

内 痔

Nèi Zhì

Definition: Internal hemorrhoid is characterized by intrahemorrhoidal venous plexus dilation above the dentate line and below the rectal mucosa, forming soft varicose veins, with bleeding in stools, prolapse of the venous mass, anal discomfort, etc. In Chinese medicine, internal hemorrhoid is referred to as nei zhi.

Pathogenesis: Internal hemorrhoid is usually caused by sitting for long periods of time, standing, walking, constipation, diarrhea, inappropriate diet, feng, dryness, shi, stasis, etc.

Treatments Based on CM Diagnosis

Internal Treatments

For stages 1 and 2, infections, seniors, and those cases not indicated for surgery.

(1) Feng Attacking the Rectum

Zheng: Blood in stools, dripping or bleeding, bright red blood, itchiness, red tongue, thin white or yellow tai, floating fast pulse.

Treatment method: Clearing heat, cooling blood, and driving out feng.

Formula: Liang xue di huang tang.

(2) Shi Heat Descending

Zheng: Blood in stools is bright red and of a large amount, prolapse of the venous mass, retractable, burning sensation in anus, red tongue, thin yellow greasy tai, stringy fast pulse.

Treatment method: Clearing heat, diuresis, and hemostasis.

Formula: Zang lian wan.

(3) Qi Stagnation Blood Stasis

Zheng: Prolapse of the venous mass, embedded, anal canal retrenching, distending pain, embolism, thrombus, edema, pain upon touching, dark tongue, white or yellow tai, stringy thin uneven pulse.

Treatment method: Clearing heat and diuresis, driving out feng and moving the blood.

Formula: Zhi tong ru shen tang.

(4) Pi Deficiency and Qi Descending

Zheng: Anus tenesmus, prolapse of the venous mass, hand assistance required for reposition, stool bloods bright or slightly red, pale complexion, fatigue, shortness of breath, anorexia, diarrhea, light red swollen tongue, teeth prints, thin white tai, weak pulse.

Treatment method: Strengthening qi and ascending.

Formula: Bu zhong yi qi tang.

External Treatments

(1) Wash with wu bei zi tang.
(2) Apply wu bei zi san, etc., compress.
(3) Apply zhi chuang ding suppository.
(4) Apply ku zhi san on prolapsed vein mass of bright red or purple color. Apply hui zao san on prolapsed vein mass of grey color.

External Hemorrhoid

外 痔

Wài Zhì

Definition: External hemorrhoid is characterized by extrahemorrhoidal venous plexus dilation below the dentate line, varicose veins, vein rupture, recurrent inflammation, bleeding in stools, tenesmus, pain, etc. In Chinese medicine, external hemorrhoid is referred to as wai zhi.

Pathogenesis: External hemorrhoid is usually caused by anal injury, recurrent nei zhi, shi, heat, stasis, labor, etc.

Treatments Based on CM Diagnosis

Internal Treatments

(1) Shi Heat Descending

Zheng: Ellipse- or long-shaped soft mass below the dentate line, worsens during bowel movement or squatting, dark purple color, not retracting after bowel movement, tenesmus, hotness, pain, exudes fluid, constipation or diarrhea, red tongue, yellow greasy tai, slippery fast pulse.

Treatment method: Clearing heat and removing shi, moving the blood and dispersing stasis.

Formula: Bi xie hua du tang and huo xue san yu tang.

(2) Blood Stasis Heat

Zheng: Extrahemorrhoidal vein rupture, clots, protruding venous mass, swelling, severe pain, tenesmus, hard nodules, dark purple, constipation, thirst, vexation, purple tongue, light yellow tai, stringy uneven pulse.

Treatment method: Clearing heat and cooling the blood, reducing swelling and stopping pain.

Formula: Liang xue di huang tang.

External Treatments

(1) Wash with ku shen tang.
(2) Compress with huang lian gao.

Mixed Hemorrhoid

混 合 痔

Hùn Hé Zhì

Definition: Mixed hemorrhoid is characterized by dilations of both the intrahemorrhoidal and extrahemorrhoidal venous plexus, combining with signs and symptoms of both internal hemorrhoid and external hemorrhoid. In Chinese medicine, mixed hemorrhoid is referred to as hun he zhi.

Pathogenesis: Mixed hemorrhoid is usually caused by recurrent internal hemorrhoid, labor, over-exertion, stasis, etc.

Treatments Based on CM Diagnosis

Internal Treatment

If the condition is not severe, refer to the Internal Treatments for internal hemorrhoid.

External Treatments

(1) Wash with ku shen tang.
(2) Compress with huang lian gao.

Anal Sinusitis

肛 隐 窝 炎

Gāng Yǐn Wō Yán

Definition: Anal sinusitis is characterized by discomfort around the anus, pain during bowel movement, short sharp pain without bowel movement, pain radiating to the thigh, constipation, mucus in stools, blood in stools, itchiness, etc. In Chinese medicine, anal sinusitis is referred to as gang yin wo yan.

Pathogenesis: Anal sinusitis is usually caused by alcohol, spicy foods, worms, shi, heat, constipation, etc.

Treatments Based on CM Diagnosis

Internal Treatment

Shi Heat Descending

Zheng: Tenesmus, anal discomfort, hot sensation, stabbing pain, worsens during bowel movement, mucus in stool, anal shi itchy, dry mouth, constipation, yellow greasy tai, slippery fast pulse.

Treatment method: Clearing heat and diuresis.

Formula: Zhi tong ru shen tang or liang xue di huang tang.

External Treatments

(1) Wash with ku shen tang.
(2) Zhi chuang ding.
(3) Surgery.

Anal Fissure

肛 裂

Gāng Liè

Definition: Anal fissure is characterized by anal pain during bowel movement, paroxysmal lancinating or hot pain which recedes after defecation, severe pain again due to sphincter spasm, anal skin splits, ulceration, triggered by coughing and sneezing, pain radiating to the pelvis and legs, blood in stools, constipation, etc. In Chinese medicine, anal fissure is referred to as gang lie.

Pathogenesis: Anal fissure is usually caused by yin deficiency, heat, shi, toxins, etc.

Based on the stages, it is divided into two classes:

(1) Early gang lie.
(2) Late gang lie.

Treatments Based on CM Diagnosis

Internal Treatments

(1) Blood Heat and Intestine Zao

Zheng: Defecating once every two to three days, hard dry stools, pain during defecation, blood in stools, split skin is bright red, abdominal distension, yellow urine, red tongue, stringy fast pulse.

Treatment method: Clearing heat, moisturing the intestine, and relaxing the bowel.

Formula: Liang xue di huang tang and pi yue ma ren wan.

(2) Yin Deficiency

Zheng: Constipation, defecating once every several days, pain during defecation, blood in stools, split skin is deep red, dry mouth, vexation, red tongue, little or no tai, thin fast pulse.

Treatment method: Nourishing yin, clearing heat, and moisturing the intestine.

Formula: Run chang tang.

External Treatments

(1) New gang lie: Sheng ji yu hong gao or huang lian gao.
(2) Old gang lie: First use qi san dan, then huang lian gao.
(3) Surgery.

Perianal Subcutaneous Abscess

肛 痈

Gāng Yōng

Definition: Perianal subcutaneous abscess is characterized by acute onset of anal swelling, severe pain, nodules, fever, listlessness, constipation, pyogenesis after five to seven days, forming fistula after diabrosis, etc. In Chinese medicine, perianal subcutaneous abscess is referred to as gang yong.

Pathogenesis: Perianal subcutaneous abscess is usually caused by fat, spicy foods, alcohol, shi, heat, toxins, zang deficiency, etc.

Treatments Based on CM Diagnosis

Internal Treatments

(1) Heat Toxins

Zheng: Sudden swelling and pain in the anal area, progressing, aversion to cold, fever, constipation, yellow urine, red, hard and hot anal area, red tongue, thin yellow tai, fast pulse.

Treatment method: Clearing heat, detoxifying, and diuresis.

Formula: Huang lian jie du tang and long dan xie gan tang.

(2) Yin Deficiency and Toxin Attack

Zheng: Anal pain, skin is dark red, pyogenesis takes a long time, pus is dilute, ulceration is difficult to heal, hectic fever in the afternoon, vexation, dry mouth, night sweats, red tongue, little tai, thin fast pulse.

Treatment method: Nourishing yin, clearing heat, and detoxifying.

Formula: Qing hao bie jia tang and san miao wan.

External Treatments

(1) For heat toxin zheng, use jin huang gao or huang lian gao.
(2) For yin deficiency zheng, use chong he gao.
(3) Pyogenesis: Surgery.

Anal Fistula

肛 瘘

Gāng Lòu

Definition: Anal fistula is characterized by recurrent or continuous exudation of pus, pain, itchiness around the anus area, fistula connecting to the rectum, difficulty healing, etc. Based on the number of openings and the layout of the fistula, it is divided into simple gang lou and complex gang lou. In Chinese medicine, anal fistula is referred to as gang lou.

Pathogenesis: Anal fistula is usually caused by gang yong, fei pi deficiency, toxins, etc.

Treatments Based on CM Diagnosis

Internal Treatments

(1) Shi Heat

Zheng: Frequent exudation of thick pus around the anus, anal distending pain, hot sensation, diabrosis opening has a thread-like object connected to the inside of the anus, red tongue, yellow tai, stringy slippery pulse.

Treatment method: Clearing heat and diuresis.

Formula: Er miao wan and bi xie shen shi tang.

(2) Yin Deficiency

Zheng: Diabrosis around the anus, sunken opening, fistula cannot be felt, pus is dilute, hectic fever, night sweats, vexation, dry mouth, red tongue, little tai, thin fast pulse.

Treatment method: Nourishing yin and clearing heat.

Formula: Qing hao bie jia tang.

External Treatments

(1) Thread-drawing method.
(2) Incision method.
(3) Combination method.

Anorectal Prolapse

脱 肛

Tuō Gāng

Definition: Anorectal prolapse is characterized by recurrent prolapse of the rectum and rectal mucosa, incomplete and unsmooth bowel movement, tenesmus, ache, distension, swelling, ulceration, hemorrhage, itchiness, etc. In Chinese medicine, anorectal prolapse is referred to as tuo gang.

Pathogenesis: Anorectal prolapse is usually caused by qi and blood deficiency, chronic diarrhea, constipation, chronic cough, etc.

Treatments Based on CM Diagnosis

Internal Treatments

(1) Pi Deficiency

Zheng: Prolapse of mass of rectum occurs during bowel movement, varying degrees, area is light red, tenesmus, blood in stools, fatigue, anorexia, dizziness, tinnitus, soreness in the waist and knees, light red tongue, thin white tai, weak pulse.

Treatment method: Strengthening qi and ascending, constringent and arresting prolapsed mass.

Formula: Bu zhong yi qi tang.

(2) Shi Heat

Zheng: Prolapse of mass of rectum occurs, area is purple-dark red, ulceration, tenesmus, hot sensation, red tongue, yellow greasy tai, stringy fast pulse.

Treatment method: Clearing heat and diuresis.

Formula: Bi xie shen shi tang.

External Treatments

(1) Wash with ku shen tang.
(2) Compress with wu bei zi san.

Rectal Polyp

息 肉 痔

Xī Ròu Zhì

Definition: Rectal polyp is characterized by neoplasm on the rectal mucosa, with no symptoms in the early stage, and possible symptoms as it progresses. Some polyps may prolapse during defecation. Other symptoms are discomfort during bowel movement, tenesmus, abdominal pain, diarrhea, blood and mucus in stools, weight loss, fatigue, anemia, etc. In Chinese medicine, rectal polyp is referred to as xi rou zhi.

Pathogenesis: Rectal polyp is usually caused by shi heat, qi stagnation, blood stasis, etc.

Treatments Based on CM Diagnosis

Internal Treatments

(1) Feng Attacking the Intestine

Zheng: Bright red blood in stools, dripping blood, blood congestion in polyps, prolapse may or may not occur, red tongue, white or thin yellow tai, floating fast pulse.

Treatment method: Clearing heat and cooling the blood, driving out feng and hemostasis.

Formula: Huai jiao wan.

(2) Qi Stagnation and Blood Stasis

Zheng: Prolapse of mass of rectum occurs, non-retractable, severe pain, affected area is purple, dark, purple tongue, uneven pulse.

Treatment method: Moving the blood and removing stasis, softening hardness and dispersing nodules.

Formula: Shao fu zhu yu tang.

(3) Pi Qi Deficiency

Zheng: Prolapse of mass of rectum occurs easily, harsh surface with a little blood, relaxed anus, light tongue, thin tai, weak pulse.

Treatment method: Reinforcing the pi and wei.

Formula: Shen ling bai zhu san.

External Treatments

(1) Use alum solution enema.
(2) Surgery.

Rectal Carcinoma

锁 肛 痔

Suǒ Gāng Zhì

Definition: Rectal carcinoma is characterized by an increase in bowel movement frequency, thinning and flattening of stools, mucus in stools, hematochezia, abdominal pain, tenesmus, nodules in the rectal mucosa or anal skin, fatigue, anemia, etc. In Chinese medicine, rectal carcinoma is referred to as suo gang zhi.

Pathogenesis: Rectal carcinoma is usually caused by emotional stress, shi, heat, qi stagnation, blood stasis, toxins, pi wei disharmony, etc.

Treatments Based on CM Diagnosis

Internal Treatments

(1) Shi Heat

Zheng: Tenesmus, increase in defecation frequency, hematochezia, dark red blood, mucus in stools, red tongue, yellow greasy tai, slippery fast pulse.

Treatment method: Clearing heat and diuresis.

Formula: Huai jiao di yu wan.

(2) Qi Stagnation and Blood Stasis

Zheng: Protruding of nodule around the anus which is stone-hard, painful, refusing pressure, hematochezia, dark purple stool, tenesmus, constipation, dark purple tongue, uneven pulse.

Treatment method: Removing stasis and eliminating stagnation, clearing heat and detoxifying.

Formula: Tao hong si wu tang and shi xiao san.

(3) Qi Yin Deficiency

Zheng: Pale complexion, leanness, fatigue, diarrhea or constipation, hematochezia, dark purple blood, tenesmus, vexation, dry mouth, night sweats, dark red tongue, little tai, thin weak fast pulse.

Treatment method: Nourishing qi and yin, clearing heat and detoxifying.

Formula: Si jun zi tang and zeng ye tang.

External Treatments

(1) For ulceration, use jiu hua gao or huang lian gao.
(2) Enema with bai jiang cao and bai hua she she cao decoction.

7. Andriatrics

Acute Epididymitis

子 痈

Zǐ Yōng

Definition: Acute epididymitis is characterized by swelling and pain of the testicle or epididymis. The acute stage may see aversion to cold, fever, anorexia, bitter taste, thirst, yellow urine, constipation, etc. In Chinese medicine, acute epididymitis is referred to as zi yong.

Pathogenesis: Acute epididymitis is usually caused by shi, heat, cold, wounds, toxins, etc.

Treatments Based on CM Diagnosis

Internal Treatments

(1) Shi Heat Descending

Zheng: Swelling and pain in the testicle or epididymis, scrotum is red and swollen, wrinkling disappears, hot sensation, lower abdominal pain, pyogenesis, aversion to cold, fever, red tongue, yellow greasy tai, slippery fast pulse.

Treatment method: Clearing heat and diuresis.

Formula: Long dan xie gan tang.

(2) Toxins Descending

Zheng: Often seen in children, accompanied by mumps, swelling testicle, aversion to cold, fever, red tongue, yellow tai, fast pulse.

Treatment method: Clearing heat and detoxifying.

Formula: Pu ji xiao du yin and jin ling zi san.

(3) Qi Stagnation and Tan Accumulation

Zheng: Nodules in epididymis, swollen scrotum, mild pain, lower abdominal discomfort, thin greasy tai, slippery pulse.

Treatment method: Soothing the gan and regulating qi, dissolving tan and dispersing nodules.

Formula: Ju he wan.

(4) Yang Deficiency

Zheng: Nodules in epididymis, swollen and cold scrotum, soreness in the waist, impotence, spermatorrhea, light red tongue with teeth prints, deep thin pulse.

Treatment method: Warming the shen and driving out cold, regulating qi and dispersing nodules.

Formula: You gui wan and yang he tang.

External Treatments

(1) Acute stage: Jin huang san or yu lu san.
(2) Pyogenesis: Incision and drainage.
(3) Chronic stage: Chong he gao.

Abscess of the Scrotum

囊 痈

Náng Yōng

Definition: Abscess of the scrotum is characterized by scrotal redness, swelling, pain, alternating cold and hot, tight skin, brightness, etc. In Chinese medicine, abscess of the scrotum is referred to as nang yong.

Pathogenesis: Abscess of the scrotum is usually caused by shi, toxins, wounds, inappropriate diet, heat, etc.

Treatments Based on CM Diagnosis

Internal Treatments

(1) Gan Shi Heat

Zheng: Scrotal redness, swelling, hot sensation, descending and pressing pain, swelling and pain in groin lymph nodes, pyogenesis, local swelling pain, throbbing pain, undulatory feeling upon pressing, fever, dry mouth, fondness for cold drinks, yellow urine, deep red tongue, yellow greasy or dry tai, stringy fast tight pulse.

Treatment method: Clearing heat, detoxifying, and diuresis.

Formula: Xie re tang.

(2) Gan Shen Yin Deficiency

Zheng: After pus is released, dry mouth, night sweats, fatigue, soreness in the waist and knees, red tongue, little tai, greasy root, thin fast pulse.

Treatment method: Regulating the gan and replenishing the shen, clearing heat and diuresis.

Formula: Zi yin chu shi tang.

External Treatments

(1) Initial stage: Yu lu gao and jin huang gao.
(2) Pyogenic stage: Incision drainage.

Tuberculosis of the Epididymis

子 痰

Zǐ Tán

Definition: Tuberculosis of the epididymis is characterized by chronic gradual increase in size of the epididymis, no obvious pain, no fever. Epididymis may stick to scrotum skin. After diabrosis exudates dilute, may form sinuses, etc. In Chinese medicine, tuberculosis of the epididymis is referred to as zi tan.

Pathogenesis: Tuberculosis of the epididymis is usually caused by gan shen deficiency, phlegm, heat, stasis, etc.

Treatments Based on CM Diagnosis

Internal Treatments

(1) Shi Tan Accumulation

Zheng: Swelling of the epididymis which is hard and experiences dull pain, light tongue, thin tai, slippery pulse.

Treatment method: Warming channels and opening collaterals, resolving tan and removing shi.

Formula: Yang he tang and xiao jin dan.

(2) Yin Deficiency Heat

Zheng: Epididymis is stuck to the scrotum skin, dark red, mild undulatory feeling after pyogenesis, hectic fever in the afternoon, night sweats, fatigue, flushing of the zygomatic area, leanness, red tongue, thin yellow tai, thin fast pulse.

Treatment method: Nourishing yin and clearing heat, removing shi and dissolving phlegm, draining pus and detoxifying.

Formula: Zi yin chu shi tang and tou nong san.

(3) Yang Deficiency and Tan Accumulation

Zheng: Chronic swelling of the epididymis which is hard and experiences dull pain, ulceration difficult to heal, cold extremities and body, pale complexion, soreness in the waist and knees, cold testicle, light tongue with teeth prints, thin white tai, weak pulse.

Treatment method: Replenishing the shen and warming yang, dissolving tan and dispersing nodules.

Formula: Xian tian da zao wan or you gui wan.

External Treatments

(1) Initial stage: Chong he gao.
(2) Pyogenesis stage: Incision and drainage.

Hydrocele Testis

水 疝

Shuǐ Shàn

Definition: Hydrocele testis is characterized by enlargement of the scrotum, usually a unilateral, smooth ellipse-shaped mass, which may be bright like crystal, descending, distension, discomfort, normal skin color, etc. In Chinese medicine, hydrocele testis is referred to as shui shan.

Pathogenesis: Hydrocele testis is usually caused by shen pi deficiency, genetic defects, shi, wounds, etc.

Treatments Based on CM Diagnosis

Internal Treatments

(1) Shen Qi Deficiency

Zheng: Often seen in infants and children, scrotum enlargement increases when standing or crying, bright like crystal, decreases when lying down, light tongue, thin white tai, thin slippery pulse.

Treatment method: Warming the shen and opening yang, transforming qi and moving water.

Formula: Ji sheng shen qi wan.

(2) Shi Heat Descending

Zheng: Moist and warm scrotum, pain in the testis, yellow urine, red tongue, greasy tai, fast pulse.

Treatment method: Clearing heat and diuresis.

Formula: Da fen qing yin.

(3) Shen Deficiency Cold Shi

Zheng: Chronic process, cold scrotum, skin thickened, descending, distension, discomfort, pale complexion, fatigue, soreness in the waist, weak legs, diarrhea, clear urine, light tongue, white tai, deep thin pulse.

Treatment method: Warming the shen and dispersing cold, transforming qi and moving water.

Formula: Jia wei wu ling san.

(4) Blood Stasis

Zheng: History of testis wound or tumor, presence of nodules, pain, non-transparent skin covering nodule, purple tongue, thin tai, thin uneven pulse.

Treatment method: Dissolving stasis, moving qi, and diuresis.

Formula: Huo xue san yu tang.

External Treatments

(1) For shen deficiency cold shi zheng, use xiao hui xiang, ju he, and warm compress.
(2) For shi heat zheng, soak with wu bei zi and ku fan decoction.
(3) Surgery.

Induration of the Penis

阴 茎 痰 核

Yīn Jīng Tán Hé

Definition: Induration of the penis is characterized by cord-like or patches of nodules, pain, deformation, etc. In Chinese medicine, induration of the penis is referred to as yin jing tan he.

Pathogenesis: Induration of the penis is usually caused by inappropriate diet, yin deficiency, huo, phlegm, etc.

Treatments Based on CM Diagnosis

Internal Treatments

(1) Tan Toxins

Zheng: Nodule skin color and temperature are normal, no obvious discomfort when the penis is relaxed, light tongue with teeth prints, thin white tai, soft pulse.

Treatment method: Promoting the pi and soothing the wei, dissolving tan and dispersing nodules.

Formula: Hua jian er chen wan.

(2) Yin Deficiency and Tan Huo

Zheng: Mild pain in the penis nodules, skin is slightly red, low fever, flushing in the afternoon, dysphoria with feverish sensation in the chest, palms, and soles, dry throat, tinnitus, soreness in the waist and knees, red tongue, little tai, thin fast pulse.

Treatment method: Nourishing yin and descending huo, dissolving tan and dispersing nodules.

Formula: Da bu yin wan and xiao he wan.

External Treatment

Use er bai san.

Bacterial Prostatitis

精 浊

Jīng Zhuó

Definition: Bacterial prostatitis is characterized by frequent micturition, urgency of urination, urodynia, urethra exuding sperm, dull pain or discomfort around the perineum, waist, and suprasymphysary area, etc. In Chinese medicine, bacterial prostatitis is referred to as jing zhuo.

Pathogenesis: Bacterial prostatitis is usually caused by inappropriate diet, shi heat, emotional stress, sexual strain, unclean sex, shen deficiency, etc.

Treatments Based on CM Diagnosis

Internal Treatments

(1) Qi Stagnation and Blood Stasis

Zheng: Discomfort in the lower abdomen and perineum, descending and distending pain in the testis, hematuria, hemospermia, purple tongue, ecchymosis, white yellow tai, deep uneven pulse.

Treatment method: Moving the blood and dispersing stasis.

Formula: Qian lie xian tang.

(2) Shi Heat Accumulation

Zheng: Frequent micturition, urgency of urination, urodynia, burning sensation, white exudates during urination or defecation, soreness in the perineum and waist, descending and distending pain in the testis, red tongue, yellow greasy tai, thin fast pulse.

Treatment method: Clearing heat and diuresis.

Formula: Ba zheng san or long dan xie gan tang.

(3) Yin Deficiency and Huo Flaming Up

Zheng: Soreness and weakness in the waist and knees, dizziness, insomnia, excessive dreaming, seminal emission, hemospermia, easily becoming erectile, white exudates from the urethra during urination or defecation, red tongue, little tai, thin fast pulse.

Treatment method: Replenishing the shen, nourishing yin, and clearing ministerial huo.

Formula: Zhi bo di huang tang and bi xie fen qing yin.

(4) Shen Yang Deficiency

Zheng: Dizziness, fatigue, soreness in the waist, cold knees, impotence, prospermia, white exudates from urethra on exertion, light tongue, white tai, deep thin pulse.

Treatment method: Warming the shen and arresting jing.

Formula: Jin suo gu jing wan and you gui wan.

External Treatments

For shi heat or qi stagnation and blood stasis, use the following:

(1) Jin huang san.
(2) Cong gui ta zhong tang.

Prostatic Hyperplasia

精 癃

Jīng Lóng

Definition: Prostatic hyperplasia is characterized by difficulty urinating, urine retension, etc. In Chinese medicine, prostatic hyperplasia is referred to as jing long.

Pathogenesis: Prostatic hyperplasia is usually caused by shen pi deficiency, phlegm, stasis, shi, heat, etc.

Treatments Based on CM Diagnosis

Internal Treatments

(1) Fei Heat

Zheng: Difficulty urinating or anuresis, dry throat, thirst, chest distress, respiration difficulty, cough with phlegm, red tongue, thin yellow tai, slippery fast pulse.

Treatment method: Clearing heat and dispersing the fei, opening and regulating water channels.

Formula: Huang qin qing fei yin.

(2) Shi Heat Descending

Zheng: Little urine which is of a yellow color, frequent urination, pain during urination, difficulty urinating or anuresis, lower abdominal distension, thirst but no desire to drink, fever, constipation, red tongue, yellow greasy tai, fast pulse.

Treatment method: Clearing heat, dissolving shi, and diuresis.

Formula: Ba zheng san.

(3) Middle Qi Descending

Zheng: Lower abdominal distension, difficulty urinating, incontinence, enuresis, fatigue, shortness of breath, light tongue, thin white tai, soft thin pulse.

Treatment method: Replenishing the middle jiao and reinforcing qi.

Formula: Bu zhong yi qi tang.

(4) Shen Yin Deficiency

Zheng: Frequent but difficult urination, incomplete urination, dizziness, soreness in the waist and knees, insomnia, excessive dreaming, dry throat, red tongue, yellow tai, thin fast pulse.

Treatment method: Nourishing the shen and replenishing yin.

Formula: Zhi bo di huang tang.

(5) Shen Yang Deficiency

Zheng: Weakness during urination, incontinence or enuresis, incomplete urination, pale complexion, fatigue, aversion to cold, soreness and weakness in the waist and knees, cold limbs, light tongue, white tai, deep thin pulse.

Treatment method: Nourishing the shen and warming yang, transforming qi and moving water.

Formula: Ji sheng shen qi wan.

(6) Qi Stagnation and Blood Stasis

Zheng: Urinating with effort or anuresis, distending pain in the perineum and lower abdomen, hematuresis, hemospermia, purple dark tongue with ecchymosis, white yellow tai, deep stringy thin uneven pulse.

Treatment method: Moving the blood and dissolving stasis, regulating qi and diuresis.

Formula: Dai di dang wan.

External Treatments

(1) Apply hot salt bag compress to the lower abdomen.
(2) Surgery.

8. Dermatology

Herpes Simplex

热 疮

Rè Chuāng

Definition: Herpes simplex is characterized by recurrent tightness, burning sensation, itchiness, and erythema around the mouth, lips, nose, cheeks, genitals, etc., then progressing to clusters of small blisters, etc. In Chinese medicine, herpes simplex is referred to as re chuang.

Pathogenesis: Herpes simplex is usually caused by feng heat, yin deficiency, etc.

Treatments Based on CM Diagnosis

Internal Treatments

(1) Fei Wei Heat Hyperactivity

Zheng: Clusters of vesicles, hotness, itchiness, vexation, depression, constipation, yellow urine, red tongue, yellow tai, stringy pulse.

Treatment method: Driving out feng and clearing heat.

Formula: Xin yi qing fei yin and zhu ye shi gao tang.

(2) Yin Deficiency Heat

Zheng: Recurrent, dry mouth and lips, mild fever after lunch, red tongue, thin tai, thin fast pulse.

Treatment method: Nourishing yin and clearing heat.

Formula: Zeng ye tang.

External Treatments

Zi jin ding, jin huang san, etc.

Herpes Zoster

蛇　串　疮

Shé Chuàn Chuāng

Definition: Herpes zoster is characterized by clusters of blisters which are painful and hot, etc. In Chinese medicine, herpes zoster is referred to as she chuan chuang.

Pathogenesis: Herpes zoster is usually caused by gan huo overacting, shi heat accumulating, exuding to the skin.

Treatments Based on CM Diagnosis

Internal Treatment

Zheng: Patches of belt-like erythema and papules, gradually developing into clusters of blisters of granule or green-bean size, three to five in a cluster, string-like, arranged in belt form, with normal skin in between, ulceration and infection after blisters are broken; large blisters, bloody vesicles, black scar tissue after necrosis; stabbing pain, rash, usually located around the waist, costal, chest, face, etc., areas, lasting for about two weeks, with low fever, fatigue, anorexia, red tongue, thin yellow tai, stringy fast pulse.

Treatment method: Clearing gan huo and removing shi heat.

Formula: Long dan xie gan tang.

Verruca Vulgaris

疣 目

Yóu Mù

Definition: Verruca vulgaris is characterized by a nodule of the size of a needle head or bean protruding on the skin of the back of the hand, fingers, head, face. It has a half-spherical or multiple-angled shape, pale white or yellow color, rough surface, is hard, papilliform, and may develop into multiple nodules, etc. In Chinese medicine, verruca vulgaris is referred to as you mu.

Pathogenesis: Verruca vulgaris is usually caused by feng heat toxins, shi, stasis, wounds, etc.

Treatments Based on CM Diagnosis

Internal Treatments

(1) Feng Heat and Blood Deficiency

Zheng: Bean-like nodule which is hard, rough, and yellow or red. Red tongue, thin tai, stringy fast pulse.

Treatment method: Nourishing and moving the blood, clearing heat and detoxifying.

Formula: Zhi hou fang.

(2) Shi Heat and Blood Stasis

Zheng: Loose nodule of a grey or brown color, dark red tongue, thin white tai, thin pulse.

Treatment method: Clearing shi heat and moving the blood.

Formula: Ma chi xian he ji.

External Treatments

(1) Wash with ban lan gen or ku shen decoction.
(2) Moxibustion.
(3) Acupuncture.

Verruca Plana

扁 瘊

Biǎn Hóu

Definition: Verruca plana is characterized by a smooth flat papule of needle-head size to bean size, light red, brown, or normal skin color, multiple distributed sparsely or in groups, which occur after scratching, on the face or the back of the hand, etc. In Chinese medicine, verruca plana is referred to as bian hou.

Pathogenesis: Verruca plana is usually caused by scratching, wounds, heat toxins, stasis, etc.

Treatments Based on CM Diagnosis

Internal Treatments

(1) Heat Toxin Accumulation

Zheng: Multiple light red papules, dry mouth, lack of thirst, fever, constipation, yellow urine, red tongue, greasy white or yellow tai, slippery fast pulse.

Treatment method: Clearing heat and detoxifying.

Formula: Ma chi xian he ji.

(2) Heat Stasis

Zheng: Chronic process, yellow-brown or dark red papule, vexation, dark red tongue, thin white tai, deep relaxed pulse.

Treatment method: Clearing heat, moving blood, and dissolving stasis.

Formula: Tao hong si wu tang.

External Treatments

(1) Wash with ban lan gen or ku shen decoction.
(2) Ya dan zi ren you.

Impetigo

黄　水　疮

Huáng Shuǐ Chuāng

Definition: Impetigo is characterized by superficial pustules and crust on the skin. It is contagious and auto-inoculating, often occurs in summer or fall, and is seen in childcare centers, kindergartens, etc. In Chinese medicine, impetigo is referred to as huang shui chuang.

Pathogenesis: Impetigo is usually caused by shi heat, summer heat, asthenia, sweat, etc.

Treatments Based on CM Diagnosis

Internal Treatments

(1) Summer Shi Heat

Zheng: Dense pustules yellow in color, while the surrounding areas are red. Bright red ulcerated area, dry mouth, constipation, yellow urine, red tongue, yellow greasy tai, soft slippery fast pulse.

Treatment method: Clearing summer heat, diuresis, and detoxifying.

Formula: Qing shu tang.

(2) Pi Deficiency and Shi Accumulation

Zheng: Sparse pustules light white or yellow in color, light red ulcerated area, anorexia, diarrhea, light tongue, thin slight greasy tai, soft thin pulse.

Treatment method: Promoting the pi and seeping shi.

Formula: Shen ling bai zhu san.

External Treatments

(1) Qing dai san.
(2) Dian dao san.
(3) For thick crust, use liu huang ruan gao or hong you gao, and jiu yi dan.

White Ringworm

白 秃 疮

Bái Tū Chuāng

Definition: White ringworm is characterized by round or irregular-shaped grey-white squames on the scalp, dry hair without luster, broken hair, hair loss, itchiness, often affecting the vertex and occiput, no scar after recovery, etc. In Chinese medicine, white ringworm is referred to as bai tu chuang.

Pathogenesis: White ringworm is usually caused by feng and heat attacks, pi wei shi heat, unfavorable living conditions, inappropriate activities, etc.

Treatments Based on CM Diagnosis

Internal Treatment

Feng Shi Accumulation

Zheng: Large extent of the skin is affected, itchiness, exudates, broken hair and hair loss, white patches, yellow scabs, thickened skin, fissures, blisters, ulceration, thin greasy tai, soft pulse.

Treatment method: Clearing heat and removing shi, eliminating feng and reducing itching.

Formula: Xiao feng san and ku shen tang.

288

External Treatments

(1) Haircut.
(2) Wash head with 0.5% ming fan solution or warm soap solution.
(3) Change once a day.
(4) One week later, pull out the hairs when they are loose.
(5) Repeat the above for three weeks.

Favus

肥 疮

Féi Chuāng

Definition: Favus is characterized by a yellow thick sticky crust dipped in the center and raised at the edge, brittle, ulcerated under the crust, starting from the vertex and may spread to the entire head, dry hair without luster, itchiness, and may cause permanent baldness. In Chinese medicine, favus is referred to as fei chuang.

Pathogenesis: Favus is usually caused by pi wei shi heat, toxins, dirty hands touching the head, unclean pillows, unclean hairdressing tools, etc.

Treatments Based on CM Diagnosis

Internal Treatments

Feng Shi Accumulation

Zheng: Large extent of the skin is affected, itchiness, exudates, broken hair and hair loss, white patches, yellow scabs, thickened skin, fissures, blisters, ulceration, thin greasy tai, soft pulse.

Treatment method: Clearing heat and removing shi, eliminating feng and reducing itching.

Formula: Xiao feng san and ku shen tang.

External Treatments

(1) Haircut.
(2) Wash head with 0.5% ming fan solution or warm soap solution.
(3) Change once a day.
(4) One week later, pull out the hairs when they are loose.
(5) Repeat the above for three weeks.

Tinea Manuum

鹅 掌 风

É Zhǎng Fēng

Definition: Tinea manuum is characterized by blisters, keratinization, and desquamation on the palm or fingers of the hand, itchiness, thickened skin, dryness, fissures, pain, dysfunction, etc. In Chinese medicine, tinea manuum is referred to as e zhang feng.

Pathogenesis: Tinea manuum is usually caused by shi, heat, dryness, blood deficiency, etc.

Treatments Based on CM Diagnosis

External Treatments

(1) Redness and moisture: Use pi zhi gao.
(2) Blisters: Use No. 1 or No. 2 xuan yao shui.
(3) Roughness and fissures: Feng you gao, fumigation therapy, etc.

Dermatophytosis

脚 湿 气

Jiǎo Shī Qì

Definition: Dermatophytosis is characterized by itchiness, ulceration, pain, blisters, exudates at the toes or sole, etc. In Chinese medicine, dermatophytosis is referred to as jiao shi qi.

Pathogenesis: Dermatophytosis is usually caused by shi, heat, sharing feet basins, shoes, ponds, etc.

Treatments Based on CM Diagnosis

Internal Treatment

Shi Heat Descending

Zheng: Foot ulceration, exuding foul-smelling fluid or pus, swelling to the ankle, or red thread grows upward, enlarged hip lymph nodes, chills, fever, red tongue, yellow greasy tai, slippery fast pulse.

Treatment method: Clearing heat, dissolving shi, and detoxifying.

Formula: Wu shen tang, bi xie hua du tang, long dan xie gan tang, etc.

External Treatments

(1) Desquamation and blisters: Use fu fang tu jin pi ding.
(2) Desquamation and dryness or fissures: Xiong huang gao.

(3) Pyogenesis: Qing dai gao.
(4) Ulceration: Soak in ban zhi lian decoction for 15 min, then apply pi zhi gao.
(5) For acute reticular lymphangitis and acute superficial lymphangitis, see related chapters.

Onychomycosis

灰 指 甲

Huī Zhǐ Jiǎ

Definition: Onychomycosis is characterized by nails losing luster, thickening, deforming, becoming grey, uneven, damaged, etc. In Chinese medicine onychomycosis is referred to as hui zhi jia.

Pathogenesis: Onychomycosis is usually caused by tinea manuum, dermatophytosis, etc.

Treatments Based on CM Diagnosis

External Treatments

Use fu fang tu jin pi ding, once a day, for 10 min each time.

Tinea Corporis

园 癣

Yuán Xuǎn

Definition: Tinea corporis is characterized by papules, developing into round macules with clear edges, about 1 cm or larger, itchy, with red papules along the edge and surrounding areas, blisters, squames, scabs, affecting the face, body, limbs, etc. In Chinese medicine, tinea corporis is referred to as yuan xuan.

Pathogenesis: Tinea corporis is usually caused by feng shi heat toxins, contact with unclean objects, etc.

Treatments Based on CM Diagnosis

External Treatments

Use dian dao san.

Dermatomycosis Microsporina

紫 白 癜 风

Zǐ Bái Diàn Fēng

Definition: Dermatomycosis microsporina is characterized by round or irregular-shaped macules which vary in size, are slightly red, purple, yellow, brown or grey-white, mildly itchy, squamous, affecting the neck, chest, back, shoulders, armpits, lower body, and may spread all over the body, relieved in winter and worse in summer, etc. In Chinese medicine, dermatomycosis microsporina is referred to as zi bai dian feng.

Pathogenesis: Dermatomycosis microsporina is usually caused by sweat, feng, shi toxins, etc.

Treatments Based on CM Diagnosis

External Treatments

Use mi tuo seng san, 10% tu jin pi ding.

Scabies

疥 疮

Jiè Chuāng

Definition: Scabies is characterized by small red papules, papulo-vesicles, small blisters, nodules, tunnels, and scabs, severe itchiness at night, with grey-white, slightly dark, or normal-colored tunnels where sarcoptic mites can be found. In Chinese medicine, scabies is referred to as jie chuang.

Pathogenesis: Scabies is usually caused by contact with sarcoptic mite-infected clothes, blankets, utensils, shi heat, etc.

Treatments Based on CM Diagnosis

Internal Treatment

Shi Heat Toxins

Zheng: Many blisters, papulo-vesicles, thin walls, plenty of fluid, exuding oily fluid, ulcerating, pustular, red thread-like areas, swollen lymph nodes, red tongue, yellow greasy tai, fast slippery pulse.

Treatment method: Clearing heat, dissolving shi, and detoxifying.

Formula: Huang lian jie du tang and wu wei xiao du yin.

External Treatments

Use 5 to 20% liu huang ointment.

Insect Dermatitis

虫 咬 皮 炎

Chóng Yǎo Pí Yán

Definition: Insect dermatitis is characterized by papules, petechiae, urticaria, erythema, papulo-vesicles, blisters, distributed disparsely or in groups, ulceration, itchiness, pain, or accompanied by fever, aversion to cold, headache, nausea, chest distress, breathing difficulty, etc. Different insects may cause different clinical signs and symptoms. In Chinese medicine, insect dermatitis is referred to as chong yao pi yan.

Pathogenesis: Insect dermatitis is usually caused by insect bites, contact with insect toxins, contact with toxic hairs and thorns, etc.

Treatments Based on CM Diagnosis

Internal Treatments

Heat Toxins

Zheng: Large red area, swelling, blisters, ecchymosis, enlarged lymph nodes, aversion to cold, fever, nausea, chest distress, red tongue, yellow tai, fast pulse.

Treatment method: Clearing heat and detoxifying.

Formula: Wu wei xiao du yin.

External Treatments

(1) Use 1% bo he san huang xi ji.
(2) For secondary infections, use qing dai gao.

Contact Dermatitis

接 触 性 皮 炎

Jiē Chù Xìng Pí Yán

Definition: Contact dermatitis is characterized by erythema, swelling, papules, blisters, bulla, ulceration, exudates, etc., after coming into contact with some materials. Different materials may cause different reactions. In Chinese medicine, contact dermatitis is referred to as jie chu xing pi yan.

Pathogenesis: Contact dermatitis is usually caused by contact with some materials such as chemicals and plants.

Treatments Based on CM Diagnosis

Internal Treatments

(1) Heat Shi Toxins

Zheng: Rapid onset, bright red skin, swelling, blisters, bulla, ulceration after rupture, exudates, hotness, itchiness, fever, thirst, constipation, yellow urine, red tongue, light yellow tai, stringy slippery fast pulse.

Treatment method: Clearing heat and eliminating shi, cooling the blood and detoxifying.

Formula: Long dan xie gan tang.

(2) Blood Deficiency and Feng Zao

Zheng: Recurrent process, skin is thickened and dry, squames, moss-like change, severe itchiness, scratch marks, scabs, light red tongue, thin tai, stringy thin fast pulse.

Treatment method: Clearing heat and driving out feng, nourishing the blood and moisturing dryness.

Formula: Xiao feng san.

External Treatments

(1) For flushing and papules, use san huang xi ji.
(2) For swelling, ulceration, and exudates, use pu gong ying or ye ju hua 30 g, or sang ye 10 g, sheng gan cao 15 g, decoction wash and compress.
(3) For ulceration and scabs, use qing dai gao.

Eczema

湿 疮

Shī Chuāng

Definition: Eczema is characterized by itchiness, ulceration, erosion, scabs, and other various forms of skin damage. In Chinese medicine, eczema is referred to as shi chuang.

Pathogenesis: Eczema is usually caused by feng, shi, heat, and other pathogenic factors accumulated in the skin.

Treatments Based on CM Diagnosis

Internal Treatments

(1) Shi Heat Accumulation

Zheng: Sudden onset of the disease with pimples, papules, erythema, red blisters, foul-smelling and sticky exudates, yellow urine, constipation, red tongue, yellow greasy tai, slippery fast pulse.

Treatment method: Clearing heat and cooling the blood, removing shi and stopping itchiness.

Formula: Long dan xie gan tang.

(2) Shi Outweighing Heat

Zheng: Chronic process, papules, papulo-vesicles, excessive fluid, fatigue, anorexia, diarrhea, clear urine, light tongue, white greasy tai, stringy slippery pulse.

Treatment method: Promoting the pi, diuresis, and clearing heat.

Formula: Chu shi wei ling tang.

(3) Blood Deficiency and Feng Zao

Zheng: Chronic process, recurrent, dark pimples and papules, thickness, infiltration, moss-like changes, pigmentation, scabs, desquamation, fatigue, soreness in the waist, weak limbs, light red tongue, thin tai, soft thin weak pulse.

Treatment method: Nourishing the blood and driving out feng, clearing heat and diuresis.

Formula: Si wu tang and bi xie shen shi tang.

Acupuncture Treatments

Points: Qu chi, xue hai, jian yu, huan tiao, he gu, du channel, wei zhong, etc.

External Treatments

(1) For the acute stage with plenty of exudates, use 10% huang bo solution or pu gong ying 30 g and ye ju hua 15 g. As exudates decrease, use qing dai san.
(2) For the subacute stage, use san huang xi ji.
(3) For the chronic stage, use qing dai gao.

Infantile Eczema

婴 儿 湿 疮

Yīng Ér Shī Chuāng

Definition: Infantile eczema is characterized by erythema, papules, blisters, or ulcerations on the face, forehead, scalp, neck, shoulders, or all over the body, swelling lymph nodes, fever, anorexia, constipation, itchiness, vexation, crying, restlessness, often seen in one- to two-year-old infants. In Chinese medicine, infantile eczema is referred to as ying er shi.

Pathogenesis: Infantile eczema is usually caused by a weak constitution, fetal huo, shi heat, feng, indigestion, allergy, contact with clothing, soap water, etc.

Treatments Based on CM Diagnosis

Internal Treatments

(1) Fetal Huo and Shi Heat

Zheng: Flushed skin, erythema, blisters, itchiness, exudates, yellow fluids, ulceration, yellow scab, constipation, yellow urine, red tongue, yellow greasy tai, slippery fast pulse.

Treatment method: Cooling the blood, diuresis, and clearing huo.

Formula: Xiao feng dao chi tang.

(2) Pi Deficiency and Shi Accumulation

Zheng: Skin starts with a dark color, then develops blisters, itchiness, scabs from scratching, indigestion, diarrhea, light tongue, white greasy tai, relaxed pulse.

Treatment method: Promoting the pi and diuresis.

Formula: Xiao er hua shi tang.

External Treatments

(1) For the seborrheic and wet types, wash with sheng di yu, huang bo decoction, then apply qing dai gao.
(2) For the dry type, use san huang xi ji.

Dermatitis Medicamentosa

药 毒

Yào Dú

Definition: Dermatitis medicamentosa is characterized by urticaria, measles, scarlet fever, multiple erythema, eczema, desquamation dermatitis, or bulla, with itchiness, hotness, fever, fatigue, anorexia, constipation, yellow urine, etc. In Chinese medicine, dermatitis medicamentosa is referred to as yao du.

Pathogenesis: Dermatitis medicamentosa is usually caused by ingestion of, injection with, or contact with medications.

Treatments Based on CM Diagnosis

Internal Treatments

(1) Shi Toxins on the Skin

Zheng: Erythema, blisters, ulceration, exudates, desquamation, severe itchiness, vexation, dry mouth, constipation, yellow urine, fever, red tongue, thin white or yellow tai, slippery fast pulse.

Treatment method: Clearing heat, diuresis, and detoxifying.

Formula: Bi xie shen shi tang.

(2) Heat Toxins in the Ying

Zheng: Bright red or purple-red rash, purpura, bloody vesicles, high fever, coma, dry lips, thirst but no desire to drink, constipation, yellow and scanty urine, deep red tongue, little tai, strong fast pulse.

Treatment method: Clearing the ying and detoxifying.

Formula: Qing ying tang.

(3) Qi Yin Deficiency

Zheng: Rash recedes, low fever, thirst, fatigue, shortness of breath, constipation, yellow urine, red tongue, little tai, thin fast pulse.

Treatment method: Strengthening qi, nourishing yin, and clearing heat.

Formula: Zeng ye tang and yi wei tang.

External Treatments

(1) For general situations, use san huang xi ji.
(2) For widespread areas, use qing dai san.
(3) For the desquamation infiltration stage, use qing dai san.

Urticaria

癮 疹

Yǐn Zhěn

Definition: Urticaria is characterized by red or pale evanescent wheals which are itchy, move around, occur on and off, and do not leave scars afterwards, etc. In Chinese medicine, urticaria is referred to as yin zhen.

Pathogenesis: Urticaria is usually caused by qi and blood deficiency, feng, cold, heat, shi, emotional stress, etc.

Treatments Based on CM Diagnosis

Internal Treatments

(1) Feng Heat Attack

Zheng: Wheals are bright red, hot, severely itchy, fever, aversion to cold, sore throat, worsening on contact with heat, red tongue, thin white or yellow tai, floating fast pulse.

Treatment method: Driving out feng and clearing heat.

Formula: Xiao feng san.

(2) Feng Cold Attack

Zheng: Wheals are white, worsening on contact with cold, and relieved by warmth, no thirst, light tongue, white tai, floating tight pulse.

Treatment method: Driving out feng and dispersing cold.

Formula: Gui zhi tang.

(3) Blood Deficiency and Feng Zao

Zheng: Recurrent wheals, chronic process, worsening in the afternoon and at night, vexation, fast temper, dry mouth, warmth in the palms and soles, red tongue, little tai, deep thin pulse.

Treatment method: Nourishing the blood, driving out feng, and moisturing dryness.

Formula: Ba zhen tang

External Treatments

Wash with two or three of the following: Xiang zhang mu, can sha, lu cao, cang er cao, ling xiao hua, ai ye, dong gua pi decoction.

Neurodermatitis

牛 皮 癣

Niú Pí Xuǎn

Definition: Neurodermatitis is characterized by round or multi-angled flat papules, itchiness, skin after scratching becomes ox-neck-like, thick, hard, easily forming moss, etc. In Chinese medicine, neurodermatitis is referred to as niu pi xuan.

Pathogenesis: Neurodermatitis is usually caused by feng, shi, heat, yin and blood deficiency, emotional stress, over-exertion, etc.

Treatments Based on CM Diagnosis

Internal Treatments

(1) Gan Huo

Zheng: Red skin, vexation, fast temper, insomnia, excessive dreaming, dizziness, palpitation, bitter mouth, dry throat, red tongue edge, stringy pulse.

Treatment method: Clearing the gan and purging huo.

Formula: Long dan xie gan tang.

(2) Feng Shi Accumulation

Zheng: Skin has light brown macules, is thick, rough, and severely itchy, especially at night. Thin white or greasy tai, soft hesitant pulse.

Treatment method: Driving out feng and diuresis.

Formula: Xiao feng san.

(3) Blood Deficiency and Feng Zao

Zheng: Pale skin like withered wood, thick and rough as ox skin, palpitation, insomnia, amnesia, irregular menstruation, light tongue, thin tai, deep thin pulse.

Treatment method: Nourishing the blood, driving out feng, and moisturing dryness.

Formula: Si wu xiao feng yin.

External Treatments

(1) Feng shi heat: San huang xi ji.
(2) Blood deficiency and feng zao: feng you gao.

Pruritus Cutis

皮 肤 瘙 痒 症

Pí Fū Sào Yǎng Zhèng

Definition: Pruritus cutis is characterized by severe itchiness of the skin, worsening at night, continuous and strong scratching until the skin is broken and painful, leaving scratching marks, scars, thickening of the skin, lichenification, etc. In Chinese medicine, pruritus cutis is referred to as pi fu sao yang zheng.

Pathogenesis: Pruritus cutis is usually caused by feng heat or blood heat accumulating in the skin, blocking the channels, or blood deficiency resulting in gan hyperactivity, leading to feng and dryness, etc.

Treatments Based on CM Diagnosis

Internal Treatments

(1) Feng Blood Heat

Zheng: Often seen in young people, new outbreak, thick bedding and clothes may trigger or worsen the situation, red tongue, thin yellow tai, slippery fast pulse.

Treatment method: Driving out feng, clearing heat, and cooling the blood.

Formula: Qing feng san.

(2) Blood Deficiency and Gan Hyperactivity

Zheng: Often seen in old people, chronic itchiness, with scratching marks, thickened skin, emotional disturbances may trigger or worsen the situation, mild dim colored tongue, thin tai, thin fast pulse.

Treatment method: Nourishing the blood and suppressing the gan, driving out feng and clearing dryness.

Formula: Di huang yin zi.

Pityriasis Rosea

风 热 疮

Fēng Rè Chuāng

Definition: Pityriasis rosea is characterized by a light red or yellow-red squamous nail-sized macule (mother macule) on the body trunk or limbs, and after a couple of weeks, many smaller but similar macules (baby macules) appear, itchy, with thin small wrinkles in the middle, clear zigzag edges, attached with some chaff-like squames, separate, bright red, brown, yellow, grey, brown, etc, on the chest, back, abdomen, proximal end of the limbs, neck, etc. In Chinese medicine, pityriasis rosea is referred to as feng re chuang.

Pathogenesis: Pityriasis rosea is usually caused by spicy foods, emotional stress, heat, feng, huo, etc.

Treatments Based on CM Diagnosis

Internal Treatments

(1) Feng Heat Accumulation

Zheng: Acute onset, round or ellipse-shaped light red macules, with thin and small wrinkles in the middle, covered with some chaff-like squames, vexation, thirst, constipation, light yellow urine, red tongue, white or thin yellow tai, floating fast pulse.

Treatment method: Driving out feng, clearing heat, and stopping itchiness.

Formula: Xiao feng san.

(2) Feng Heat and Blood Zao

Zheng: Bright red or purple-red macules, many chaff-like squames, severe itchiness, scratchy scabs, red tongue, little tai, stringy fast pulse.

Treatment method: Cooling the blood and clearing heat, nourishing the blood and moisturing dryness.

Formula: Liang xue xiao feng san.

External Treatments

(1) San huang xi ji or dian dao san.
(2) 5 to 10% liu huang ruan gao.
(3) Wash with the following decoction: Ku shen 30 g, she chuang zi 30 g, chuan jiao mu 12 g, ming fan 12 g.

Psoriasis

白 疕

Bái Bǐ

Definition: Psoriasis is characterized by recurrent red papules or erythema covered with multiple layers of grey dry squames, red hemorrhage spots appearing after scraping off the squames, chronic process, many variations, etc. In Chinese medicine, psoriasis is referred to as bai bi.

Pathogenesis: Psoriasis is usually caused by ying blood deficiency, feng, gan shen deficiency, blood stasis, etc.

Treatments Based on CM Diagnosis

Internal Treatments

(1) Feng Heat and Blood Zao

Zheng: Bright red papules or erythema increase continuously, bright thin film and hemorrhage spots appear after scraping off the squames, friction, wound, or puncture areas may get outbreak, vexation, thirst, constipation, yellow urine, red tongue, yellow greasy tai, stringy slippery fast pulse.

Treatment method: Clearing heat and detoxifying, cooling and moving the blood.

Formula: Xi jiao di huang tang or liang xue di huang tang.

(2) Blood Deficiency and Feng Zao

Zheng: Light red papules or erythema, some of it recedes, plenty of squames, dry mouth, constipation, light red tongue, thin white tai, thin hesitant pulse.

Treatment method: Nourishing and soothing the blood, driving out feng and moisturing dryness.

Formula: Si wu tang and xiao feng san.

(3) Blood Stasis

Zheng: Skin thickened, long-lasting dark red color, purple dark tongue with ecchymosis, uneven thin hesitant pulse.

Treatment method: Moving the blood and removing stasis.

Formula: Tao hong si wu tang.

External Treatments

(1) Niu pi xuan gao yao.
(2) No. 2 xuan yao shui or feng you gao.
(3) 10% liu huang ruan gao.

Seborrheic Dermatitis

白 屑 风

Bái Xiè Fēng

Definition: Seborrheic dermatitis is characterized by skin that is oily and itchy, with recurrent white scraps, often occuring at the scalp, face, between the eyebrows, chest, armpits, etc. Depending on the moisture of the skin, it falls into the dry type and wet type. In Chinese medicine, seborrheic dermatitis is referred to as bai xie feng.

Pathogenesis: Seborrheic dermatitis is usually caused by feng, heat, shi, yin blood deficiency, etc.

Treatments Based on CM Diagnosis

Internal Treatments

(1) Fei Wei Heat Hyperactivity

Zheng: Acute onset, red skin, exudates, ulceration, scabs, severe itchiness, vexation, thirst, constipation, red tongue, yellow tai, slippery fast pulse.

Treatment method: Clearing heat and stopping itchiness.

Formula: Pi pa qing fei yin.

(2) Pi Deficiency and Shi Accumulation

Zheng: Chronic process, light red or yellow skin, with grey squames, diarrhea, light red tongue, white greasy tai, slippery pulse.

Treatment method: Promoting the pi and diuresis.

Formula: Shen ling bai zhu san.

(3) Blood Deficiency and Feng Zao

Zheng: Dry skin, chaff-like squames, itchiness, hair dry and without luster, hair loss, red tongue, thin white tai, stringy pulse.

Treatment method: Nourishing the blood and moisturing dryness.

Formula: Dang gui yin zi.

External Treatments

(1) For the dry type on the scalp, use ce bai ye ding.
(2) For the dry type on the face, use dian dao san.
(3) For the wet type, use qing dai gao.

Acne

粉 刺

Fěn Cì

Definition: Acne is characterized by thorn-like pimples on the face, chest, back, etc., areas. When the pimples are squeezed, toothpaste-like substances may be exuded. In Chinese medicine, acne is referred to as fen ci.

Pathogenesis: Acne is usually caused by fei channel feng heat, chang wei shi heat, or pi transport dysfunction.

Treatments Based on CM Diagnosis

Internal Treatments

(1) Fei Channel Feng Heat

Zheng: Flushed complexion, hot pimples, pain, pustules, red tongue, thin yellow tai, thin fast pulse.

Treatment method: Driving out feng, dispersing the fei, and clearing heat.

Formula: Pi pa qing fei yin.

(2) Chang Wei Shi Heat

Zheng: Red pimples, swelling, pain, constipation, yellow urine, poor appetite, abdominal distension, red tongue, yellow greasy tai, slippery fast pulse.

Treatment method: Clearing heat, resolving shi, and catharsis.

Formula: Yin chen hao tang.

(3) Pi Transportation Failure

Zheng: Pimples are dark red, occur on and off, forming cysts, anorexia, diarrhea, fatigue, light tongue, white tai, soft slippery pulse.

Treatment method: Strengthening the pi and resolving shi.

Formula: Shen ling bai zhu san.

External Treatment

Use dian dao san.

Rosacea

酒 皶 鼻

Jiǔ　Zhā　Bí

Definition: Rosacea is characterized by redness, erythema, papules, pustules, etc., on the nose and surrounding areas, purple-red color, swelling, thickening, rhinophyma, etc. In Chinese medicine, rosacea is referred to as jiu zha bi.

Pathogenesis: Rosacea is usually caused by feng, cold, heat, stasis, alcohol, trichocryptosis, etc.

Treatments Based on CM Diagnosis

Internal Treatments

(1) Fei Wei Heat

Zheng: Erythema on the apex and wing of the nose, fading away upon pressing, yearn for alcohol, constipation, irregular diet, dry mouth, thirst, red tongue, thin yellow tai, stringy slippery pulse.

Treatment method: Clearing fei wei heat.

Formula: Pi pa qing fei yin.

(2) Heat Toxins in the Skin

Zheng: Erythema, papules, pustules, dilation of capillaries, hotness, dry mouth, constipation, deep red tongue, yellow tai, strong fast pulse.

Treatment method: Cooling the blood, clearing heat, and detoxifying.

Formula: Huang lian jie du tang.

(3) Qi Stagnation and Blood Stasis

Zheng: Hyperplasia of nasal tissue, nodules, dilation of capillaries, light red tongue, deep hesitant pulse.

Treatment method: Moving the blood, clearing stasis, and dispersing nodules.

Formula: Tong qiao huo xue tang.

External Treatments

(1) Erythema and papules: Dian dao san.
(2) Pustules: Si huang gao.

Alopecia Areata

油 风

Yóu Fēng

Definition: Alopecia areata is characterized by patches of hair loss, bright red scalp with luster, and may affect the eyebrows, beard, axillary hair, pubes, or even result in total hair loss, etc. In Chinese medicine, alopecia areata is referred to as you feng.

Pathogenesis: Alopecia areata is usually caused by spicy foods, emotional stress, feng, heat, wounds, qi blood deficiency, etc.

Treatments Based on CM Diagnosis

Internal Treatments

(1) Blood Heat and Feng Zao

Zheng: Sudden loss of patches of hair, occasionally itchy scalp, hot head, vexation, fast temper, restlessness, red tongue, thin yellow tai, stringy pulse.

Treatment method: Cooling the blood and calming feng, nourishing yin and protecting hair.

Formula: Si wu tang and liu wei di huang tang.

(2) Qi Stagnation and Blood Stasis

Zheng: Chronic process, headache or chest pain, hypochondriac pain that existed before hair loss, frequent nightmare, vexation, insomnia, ecchymosis on the tongue, deep thin pulse.

Treatment method: Opening orifices and moving the blood.

Formula: Tong qiao huo xue tang.

(3) Qi Blood Deficiency

Zheng: Patches of hair loss after a major disease or in the postpartum period, progressive enlargement, sparse and dry hair, easily dropping upon touching, white lips, palpitation, shortness of breath, fatigue, light tongue, thin white tai, thin weak pulse.

Treatment method: Strengthening qi and nourishing the blood.

Formula: Ba zhen tang.

(4) Gan Shen Deficiency

Zheng: Chronic process, dry yellow or grey hair, during the outbreak large patches of hair fall out or all hair falls out, dizziness, tinnitus, soreness in the waist and knees, light tongue, exfoliative tai, thin pulse.

Treatment method: Nourishing gan shen.

Formula: Qi bao mei ran dan.

External Treatments

(1) Mao jiang with vinegar.
(2) Fresh sheng jiang.
(3) 5 to 10% ban mao ding or 10% la jiao ding.

Erythema Multiforme

猫 眼 疮

Māo Yǎn Chuāng

Definition: Erythema multiforme is characterized by erythema, may be accompanied by papules, blisters, existing on the hands, feet, face, mouth, nose, and pudendum, etc. It is generally distributed symmetrically, and may be accompanied by whole body reactions. It is usually seen in young people. In Chinese medicine, erythema multiforme is referred to as mao yan chuang.

Pathogenesis: Erythema multiforme is usually caused by feng, cold, shi heat, etc., toxins.

Treatments Based on CM Diagnosis

Internal Treatments

(1) Feng Cold

Zheng: Erythema is red in color, may be accompanied by aversion to cold, cold extremities, abdominal pain, outbreak occurs or worsens in cold shi weather, and lessens or disappears in warm weather, light red tongue, white tai, soft moderate pulse.

Treatment method: Regulate ying and eliminating cold.

Formula: Gui zhi tang.

(2) Feng Shi Heat

Zheng: Erythema is a bright red, may have blisters, fever, dry mouth, constipation, yellow urine, exists all year round, may get worse in the summer, red tongue, yellow tai, slippery fast pulse.

Treatment method: Driving out feng, clearing heat, and diuresis.

Formula: Yin chen hao tang.

(3) Huo Toxins

Zheng: Sudden onset, whole body erythema, pimples, blisters, erosion, bleeding, scabs, affecting the mouth and pudendum, accompanied by aversion to cold, fever, headache, fatigue, chest pain, cough, dry and sore throat, deep red tongue, yellow tai, slippery fast pulse.

Treatment method: Clearing heat, cooling the blood, and detoxifying.

Formula: Pu ji xiao du yin.

Purpura

紫 斑

Zǐ Bān

Definition: Purpura is characterized by purple, red, or dark spots or ecchymosis under the skin. In Chinese medicine, purpura is referred to as zi ban.

Pathogenesis: Purpura is usually caused by heat toxins, yin deficiency, pi deficiency, etc.

Treatments Based on CM Diagnosis

Internal Treatments

(1) Blood Heat

Zheng: Skin has purple spots or ecchymosis, and may be accompanied by nosebleed, gingival hemorrhage, hemafecia, hematuria, fever, thirst, constipation, red tongue, yellow tai, fast pulse.

Treatment method: Clearing heat and detoxifying, cooling the blood and hemostasis.

Formula: Xi jiao di huang tang.

(2) Yin Deficiency and Huo Flaming Up

Zheng: Recurrent spots and ecchymosis on the skin, and may be accompanied by nosebleed, gingival hemorrhage, warm sensation in the palms and soles, tidal heat, flushing cheeks, red tongue, little tai, thin fast pulse.

Treatment method: Nourishing yin and suppressing huo, calming channels and hemostasis.

Formula: Qian gen san.

(3) Qi Cannot Arrest Blood

Zheng: Recurrent spots or ecchymosis on the skin, occurs on and off, fatigue, listlessness, dizziness, pale complexion, light red tongue, thin white tai, thin weak pulse.

Treatment method: Nourish qi to arrest blood.

Formula: Gui pi tang.

9. Ophthalmology

Stye

针 眼

Zhēn Yǎn

Definition: Stye is characterized by a small boil or furuncle on the palpebral margins, which looks like a wheat seed, is itchy, red, swollen, and painful. There is fever, headache, aversion to cold, etc. In Chinese medicine, stye is referred to as zhen yan.

Pathogenesis: Stye is usually caused by external feng heat, spicy and fatty food, pi wei heat toxins and deficiency, etc.

Treatments Based on CM Diagnosis

Internal Treatments

(1) Feng Heat Attack

Zheng: Initially, swelling in the eye, with mild itchiness and pain. Then a localized hard furuncle forms around the palpebral margins with pressing pain, fever, headache, red tongue, thin white tai, floating fast pulse.

Treatment method: Driving out feng and clearing heat.

Formula: Yin qiao san.

(2) Heat Toxin Attack

Zheng: Palpebral margins are red, swollen, hot, and painful with relatively large furuncles, fever, aversion to cold, dry mouth, thirst, fondness for cold drinks, constipation, yellow urine, red tongue, yellow dry tai, strong fast pulse.

Treatment method: Clearing heat, purging huo and detoxifying.

Formula: Qing wei san.

(3) Pi Wei Deficiency

Zheng: Palpebral margins are slightly red and swollen, with furuncles, mild itchiness and pain, lingering for a long time, occurring on and off, pale complexion, fatigue, anorexia, diarrhea, light red tongue, thin white tai, deep weak pulse.

Treatment method: Promoting the pi and nourishing qi, expelling toxins and draining pus.

Formula: Tuo li xiao du san.

Acupuncture Treatments

(1) Body Acupuncture

Points: Jing ming, zan zhu, si zhu kong, tong zi liao, yang bai, yu yao, tai yang, da zhui, etc.

(2) Auricular Acupuncture

Points: Mu 1, mu 2, yan, gan, dan, pang guang, xiao chang, pi, wei, etc.

Trachoma

椒 疮

Jiāo Chuāng

Definition: Trachoma is characterized by multiple red, hard granules inside the eyelids, with the size of prickly ash seeds. Slightly itchy and dry at the beginning, redness around the inner canthus with multiple small, red, needle-tip-sized granules inside the upper eyelid. The granules grow to the size of prickly ash seeds, are yellow-red or dark red, and filled with turbid serum. The granules are of different shapes with vague edges, and may merge together. It may spread to the lower eyelid. Astringent pain, photophobia, excessive gum and tears, heaviness of the eyelid, difficulty opening eyes, red vessels drop down above the black of eye, from thin vessels to patch of redness covering the black of eye, and may affect vision. In Chinese medicine, trachoma is referred to as jiao chuang.

Pathogenesis: Trachoma is usually caused by lack of eye hygiene, feng heat toxin attack, etc.

Treatments Based on CM Diagnosis

Internal Treatments

(1) Feng Heat Attack

Zheng: Eye is itchy, with astringent pain and discomfort, slightly red inside the eyelid with a small number of red granules, slightly red tongue, white tai, floating pulse.

Treatment method: Driving out feng and clearing heat.

Formula: Yin qiao san.

(2) Pi Wei Excessive Heat

Zheng: Eye is itchy, with astringent pain, excessive gum and tears, redness with many granules inside the eyelid, constipation, yellow urine, red tongue, yellow tai, fast pulse.

Treatment method: Clearing the pi and wei and dispersing feng.

Formula: Chu feng qing pi yin.

(3) Shi Heat Accumulation

Zheng: Multiple granules inside the eyelid, may be diabrotic and sticky, itchiness, astringent stabbing pain, photophobia, lachrymation, excessive sticky eye gum, red tongue, yellow greasy tai, slippery pulse.

Treatment method: Clearing heat and eliminating shi.

Formula: Qing pi yin.

(4) Blood Heat Accumulation

Zheng: Eyelid is swollen and hard, many red granules inside the eyelid, heavy eyelid, difficulty opening the eyelid, hot and stabbing pain, excessive eye gum and tears, red tongue with ecchymosis, yellow tai, strong fast pulse.

Treatment method: Cooling the blood and promoting circulation.

Formula: Gui shao hong hua san.

Acupuncture Treatments

Points: Jing ming, zan zhu, gan shu, pi shu, si bai, qu chi, feng chi, si zhu kong, etc.

Blepharoptosis

上　胞　下　垂

Shàng Bāo Xià Chuí

Definition: Blepharoptosis is characterized by drooping of the upper eyelid, covering part of or the entire pupil, and affecting the vision. It may happen in one eye or both eyes. In Chinese medicine, blepharoptosis is referred to as shang bao xia chui.

Pathogenesis: Blepharoptosis is usually caused by genetic defects, pi shen yang deficiency, yang qi descending, eyelids lacking strength, tan and shi, feng xie attack, etc.

Treatments Based on CM Diagnosis

Internal Treatments

(1) Pi Qi Deficiency

Zheng: Drooping in both the upper eyelids, chronic onset, relieved in the morning and worsens in the afternoon, progresses gradually, fatigue, anorexia, light red tongue, white tai, deep thin weak pulse.

Treatment method: Nourishing qi and ascending yang.

Formula: Bu zhong yi qi tang.

(2) Feng Tan Blockage

Zheng: Usually happens in one eye, acute onset, numbness of the eyelid, strabismus, difficulty rotating the eyeball, mydriasis, dizziness, nausea, light red tongue, white greasy tai, slippery pulse.

Treatment method: Eliminating feng and removing phlegm.

Formula: Zheng rong tang.

(3) Pi Shen Yang Deficiency

Zheng: Drooping in both the upper eyelids from a young age, weakness in lifting eyelids, raising head when looking, fatigue, aversion to cold, pale complexion, light red tongue, white tai, deep weak slow pulse.

Treatment method: Warming pi shen and strengthening yang.

Formula: Li zhong wan and you gui yin.

Acupuncture Treatments

Points: Zan zhu, yong quan, gan shu, pi shu, shen shu, shen mai, xue hai, zhong feng, yang bai, yang ling quan, zu san li.

Acute Infectious Conjunctivitis

天 行 赤 眼

Tiān Xíng Chì Yǎn

Definition: Acute infectious conjunctivitis is characterized by sudden redness of the whites of the eyes and excessive sticky eye gum. It affects both eyes, is infectious, and may affect vision. In Chinese medicine, acute infectious conjunctivitis is referred to as tian xing chi yan.

Pathogenesis: Acute infectious conjunctivitis is usually caused by epidemic pathogenic factors, or is accompanied by fei wei heat, etc.

Treatments Based on CM Diagnosis

Internal Treatments

(1) Initial Stage

Zheng: Redness of the whites of the eyes, slightly itchy and dry, not too much eye gum, no obvious whole body symptoms, light red tongue, thin white tai, floating pulse.

Treatment method: Driving out feng, dispersing pathogens, and clearing heat

Formula: Qu feng san re yin.

(2) Intermediate Stage

Zheng: Affected eyes are red, painful, and swollen, the whites of the eyes are full of redness, may be accompanied by hemorrhage, sticky eye

336

gum, headache, vexation, constipation, yellow urine, red tongue, yellow tai, fast pulse.

Treatment method: Clearing heat and detoxifying, purging huo and dispersing stagnation.

Formula: Sang bai pi tang.

(3) Recovery Stage

Zheng: The above signs and symptoms recede gradually, the redness of the whites of the eyes remain, dry and astringent eyes, occasional eye gum, dry red tongue, yellow tai, thin fast pulse.

Treatment method: Clearing heat, moisturizing the fei, and detoxifying.

Formula: Qing zao jiu fei tang.

Acupuncture Treatments

Points: He gu, qu chi, zan zhu, si zhu kong, jing ming, tong zi liao, feng chi, etc.

Chronic Conjunctivitis

白 涩 证

Bái Sè Zhèng

Definition: Chronic conjunctivitis is characterized by dryness, astringent pain, and discomfort in the eyes. There is no redness or swelling of the eyes. In Chinese medicine, chronic conjunctivitis is referred to as bai se zheng.

Pathogenesis: Chronic conjunctivitis is usually caused by feng heat attack, incomplete treatments of acute conjunctivitis, fei yin deficiency, gan shen yin deficiency, etc.

Treatments Based on CM Diagnosis

Internal Treatments

(1) Pathogenic Heat Accumulation

Zheng: Ineffective or incomplete treatments of acute conjunctivitis result in dryness and astringent pain in the eyes, light redness in the whites of the eyes, small amount of gum in the eyes, red tongue, thin yellow tai, fast pulse.

Treatment method: Clearing heat and soothing the fei.

Formula: Sang bai pi tang.

(2) Fei Yin Deficiency

Zheng: Dryness and astringent pain in the eyes, little tearing, eye fatigue after reading, blurred vision, light redness in the whites of the eyes, dry cough, little mucus, red dry tongue, white tai, thin weak pulse.

Treatment method: Replenishing yin and nourishing the fei.

Formula: Yang yin qing fei tang.

(3) Gan Shen Deficiency

Zheng: Dryness and astringent pain in the eyes, photophobia, frequent winking, blurred vision, light redness of the whites of the eyes, worsens with reading, dry mouth, soreness in the waist and knees, dizziness, tinnitus, red tongue, little tai, thin pulse.

Treatment method: Reinforcing gan shen.

Formula: Qi ju di huang tang.

Glaucoma

绿/青 风 内 障

Lù/Qīng Fēng Nèi Zhàng

Definition: In Chinese medicine, glaucoma is referred to as lu feng nei zhang and qing feng nei zhang. Lu feng nei zhang is characterized by a sudden decrease in vision, distended and hardened eyeballs, affecting the forehead and nose, increase in intraocular pressure, enlarged pupils, light green pupils, severe headache, eye pain, etc. If treatment is delayed or treated inappropriately, blindness may result. Qing feng nei zhang is characterized by no symptoms or eye distension, headache, rainbow circle around light or huo, gradual enlargement of the pupils, gradual decrease in vision, gradual decrease in vision angle, hardened eyeballs, pupil color like light blue smoke, etc. It may lead to blindness too if treatment is delayed or inappropriate.

Pathogenesis: Glaucoma is usually caused by emotional trauma, pi shi tan heat feng, over-exertion, etc.

Treatments Based on CM Diagnosis

Internal Treatments

(1) Tan Huo Feng Attacking the Eyes

Zheng: Sudden onset, headache which feels like being hit by an axe, eye pain which feels like being struck by an awl, rapid decrease in vision, ciliary hyperemia, the black of the eye is fog-like, enlarged pupil, color of pupil is light green, eyeballs harden and become stone-like, nausea, vomiting, yellow urine, constipation, red tongue, yellow greasy tai, stringy slippery fast pulse.

Treatment method: Resolving tan and calming feng, clearing heat and purging huo.

Formula: Lu feng ling yang yin and ling yang gou teng tang.

(2) Qi Stagnation and Huo Ascending

Zheng: Emotional disturbance, headache, eye distending pain, eyeball hardens, chest distension, nausea, bitter taste in the mouth, red tongue, yellow tai, stringy thin pulse.

Treatment method: Clearing heat and soothing the gan, regulating qi and descending huo.

Formula: Dan zhi xiao yao san.

(3) Yin Deficiency, Yang Overacting, and Feng Yang Ascending

Zheng: Headache and eye distending pain, blurred vision, rainbow around light and huo, vexation, insomnia, dizziness, tinnitus, red tongue, little tai, stringy thin fast pulse.

Treatment method: Nourishing yin and purging huo, suppressing the gan and putting off feng.

Formula: E jiao ji zi huang tang.

(4) Gan Shen Deficiency and Jing Blood Insufficiency

Zheng: Vision decreases gradually, vision angle narrows slowly, pupil enlarges, eyeball hardens, dryness and astringent pain in the eye, soreness in the waist and knees, light red tongue, little tai, thin pulse.

Treatment method: Reinforcing gan shen, nourishing the jing and blood.

Formula: Jia jian zhu jing wan.

Acupuncture Treatments

(1) Body Acupuncture

Points: Jing ming, zan zhu, tong zi liao, yang bai, si bai, tai bai, feng chi, yi ming, he gu, etc.

(2) Auricular Acupuncture

Points: Er jian, mu, yan, gan, dan, jiao gan, shen men, etc.

Optic Atrophy
青　盲
Qīng Máng

Definition: Optic atrophy is characterized by a gradual decrease in vision until blindness occurs without external eye symptoms. The fundus examination may see an optic disc which is pale with clear edges, and decrease in vessels. In Chinese medicine, optic atrophy is referred to as qing mang.

Pathogenesis: Optic atrophy is usually caused by gan shen deficiency, gan qi stagnation, or qi blood stasis.

Treatments Based on CM Diagnosis

Internal Treatments

(1) Gan Shen Deficiency

Zheng: Eyes look normal, vision decreases gradually until blindness occurs, dizziness, tinnitus, soreness in the waist and knees, light tongue, little tai, thin pulse.

Treatment method: Nourishing gan shen, opening channels and orifices.

Formula: Shui lun bing zhu fang.

(2) Gan Qi Stagnation

Zheng: Vision gradually decreases until blindness occurs, accompanied by emotional disturbance, dizziness, distending feeling in the eye, bitter taste in the mouth, hypochondriac pain, red tongue, white tai, stringy thin fast pulse.

Treatment method: Soothing the gan, clearing heat, and opening the sweat pores.

Formula: Dan zhi xiao yao san.

(3) Qi and Blood Stasis

Zheng: Eyes look normal, vision gradually decreases until blindness occurs or blindness occurs due to head and eye injury, headache, amnesia, dark tongue with ecchymosis, thin tai, hesitant pulse.

Treatment method: Promoting blood circulation, clearing channels, and opening orifices.

Formula: Xue fu zhu yu tang.

Acupuncture Treatments

Points: Jing ming, qiu hou, shang ming, tai yang, feng chi, gan shu, shen shu, pi shu, zhu san li, san yin jiao, etc.

10. Otology

Furuncle of the External Auditory Meatus
耳 疖
Ěr Jiē

Definition: Furuncle of the external auditory meatus is characterized by localized redness, swelling, small protrusion, severe pain within the external auditory canal. In Chinese medicine, furuncle of the external auditory meatus is referred to as er jie.

Pathogenesis: Furuncle of the external auditory meatus is usually caused by scratching, dirty water, infection, etc., which produce the heat toxins and pus, attack the skin, and lead to this disease.

Treatments Based on CM Diagnosis

Internal Treatment

Zheng: Acute onset, ear pain, pain increases when ear is stretched or pressed. One to several localized furuncles in the external auditory canal with pressing pain. May be accompanied by fever, aversion to cold, headache, red tongue, thin yellow tai, fast pulse.

Treatment method: Clearing heat, detoxifying, reducing swelling, stopping pain.

Formula: Wu wei xiao du yin.

External Treatments

(1) At the early stage, apply hot compress, alcohol ice compress, phenol glycerin drops, or a compress made from a small piece of gauze dipped in a herbal decoction. Replace once a day.

(2) When pus forms but has not broken, use three-edged needle or surgical knife to break the tip of the furuncle, let the pus out, and apply huang lian gao.

(3) When pus forms and has broken, apply huang lian ear drops, otitis ear drops, or apply a compress made from a small piece of gauze dipped in a herbal decoction.

Inflammation of the External Auditory Meatus

耳 疮

Ěr Chuāng

Definition: Inflammation of the external auditory meatus is characterized by diffuse redness, swelling, ulceration, accompanied by a small amount of pus in the external auditory canal. In Chinese medicine, inflammation of the external auditory meatus is referred to as er chuang.

Pathogenesis: Inflammation of the external auditory meatus is usually caused by scratching, wounds, dirty water, etc., which lead to feng, shi, heat toxins, or gan dan shi heat attacking the ear canal.

Treatments Based on CM Diagnosis

Internal Treatments

(1) Feng Shi Heat Toxins

Zheng: Hot sensation, itchiness, pain, diffuse redness and swelling, ulceration, in the external auditory canal, accompanied by a small amount of pus, fever, headache. Red tongue tip, thin yellow greasy tai, fast pulse.

Treatment method: Driving out feng, clearing heat, removing shi, reducing swelling.

Formula: Wu wei xiao du yin and xiao feng san.

(2) Gan Dan Shi Heat

Zheng: Diffuse redness, swelling, narrowness or closing of the external auditory canal, hot sensation, pain, ulceration, with a larger amount of pus, foul odor, tinnitus, loss of hearing, pressing pain, fever, bitter mouth, red tongue, yellow greasy tai, stringy fast pulse.

Treatment method: Clearing gan dan heat, removing shi, reducing swelling.

Formula: Long dan xie gan tang.

External Treatments

(1) At the early stage, apply huang lian ear drops, ice alcohol ear drops, three to four times a day. Or use a compress made from a small piece of gauze dipped in herbal decoction. Replace once a day.

(2) When the skin is broken, with redness, swelling, ulceration, pus, etc., use a small piece of gauze dipped in huang lian ear drops, and place on the diseased area. Replace once a day. Or apply jin huang gao, two to three times a day.

Eczema of the Ear

旋 耳 疮

Xuán Ěr Chuāng

Definition: Eczema of the ear is characterized by moisture, redness, swelling, thickness, hot sensation, itchiness, pain, ulceration, scabs, rhagades, etc., on the skin around the external auditory meatus or external ear. In severe cases, it may affect the entire auricular concha and external auditory canal. It may relapse repeatedly, and become a chronic disease. In Chinese medicine, eczema of the ear is referred to as xuan er chuang.

Pathogenesis: Eczema of the ear is usually caused by feng, shi, heat toxins, etc., attacking the skin of the ear. Toxins residing in the skin of the external ear, together with blood deficiency, lead to dryness and feng, and evolve to this disease.

Treatments Based on CM Diagnosis

This disease has both acute onset and chronic onset. It is necessary to differentiate them in clinical practice.

Internal Treatments

(1) Feng Shi Heat Toxins

Zheng: Moisture, redness, swelling, hot sensation, and itchiness around the posterior auricular sulcus, periotic skin, and auricular concha. May be accompanied by blisters, ulceration, pus exuding, pain, red tongue, yellow greasy tai, fast pulse.

348

Treatment method: Clearing shi heat, removing feng, and stopping itchiness.

Formula: Xiao feng san and bi xie shen shi tang.

(2) Blood Deficiency with Zao

Zheng: Dryness, thickness, scabs, rhagades, and itchiness of the skin around the posterior auricular sulcus, periotic skin, and auricular concha, lingering or relapsing repeatedly. May be accompanied by pale complexion, fatigue, weakness, light tongue, white tai, thin moderate pulse.

Treatment method: Nourishing the blood, reducing dryness, promoting blood circulation, and putting off feng.

Formula: Si wu xiao feng yin.

External Treatments

(1) Wash with hua jiao ye, an shu ye, tao ye, pu gong ying, ju hua decoction.
(2) For cases with severe yellowish exudates, apply qing dai san compress.
(3) For cases with severe hotness, swelling, and pain, apply san huang xi ji.
(4) For cases with pus and scabs, apply huang lian gao after pus clears.

Aural Distension

耳 胀

Ěr Zhàng

Definition: Aural distension is characterized by sudden distending pain and a feeling of fullness inside the ear, like being blocked by some object, and with hearing loss. In Chinese medicine, aural distension is referred to as er zhang.

Pathogenesis: Aural distension is usually caused by external feng heat, dan channel heat, and gan dan shi heat.

Treatments Based on CM Diagnosis

Internal Treatments

(1) Feng Heat Attack

Zheng: Acute onset of distending pain and feeling of fullness inside the ear, loss of hearing, tinnitus-like feng, ear membrane is light red or yellow and dipped, fever, aversion to cold, headache, stuffy nose with yellowish nasal discharge, red tongue tip, thin yellow tai, floating fast pulse.

Treatment method: Driving out feng, clearing heat, detoxifying, opening up the ear canal.

Formula: Yin qiao san.

(2) Dan Channel Heat

Zheng: Sudden distending pain and feeling of fullness inside the ear, like being blocked by an external object, loss of hearing, tinnitus with warm feeling, light red ear membrane, distended vessels, headache, bitter taste in the mouth, dry throat, fever, fast temper, red tongue edge, yellow tai, stringy fast pulse.

Treatment method: Clearing dan heat, moving qi, and opening up the ear canal.

Formula: Xiao chai hu tang and tong qi san.

(3) Gan Dan Shi Heat

Zheng: Distending pain and feeling of fullness inside the ear, like being blocked by an external object, loss of hearing, wave tinnitus, red ear membrane, distended vessels, headache, dizziness, fast temper, bitter taste, sticky mouth, red tongue, yellow greasy tai, stringy fast pulse.

Treatment method: Clearing gan dan heat, removing shi, and detoxifying.

Formula: Long dan xie gan tang.

External Treatments

(1) Use huang lian ear drops, ice alcohol fluid, etc., and apply to the ear two to three times a day.
(2) Use di bi ling, and apply to the nose three to four times a day.

Acupuncture Treatments

(1) Body Acupuncture

Points: Ting gong, ting hui, er men, yi feng, he gu, nei guan, etc.

(2) Auricular Acupuncture

Points: Nei er, wai er, shen men, shen shang xian, nei fen mi, fei, dan, etc.

Deafness

耳 闭

Ěr Bì

Definition: Deafness is characterized by a feeling of dull distension and fullness inside the ear, similar to being blocked by an external object, loss of hearing, lingering for a long time. In Chinese medicine, deafness is referred to as er bi.

Pathogenesis: Deafness usually develops from ineffective, delayed treatments, or relapse of acute nonsuppurative otitis media. Toxins gather inside the ear, qi and blood become stagnant, or there is pi deficiency, shi blockage, light yang descending, etc.

Treatments Based on CM Diagnosis

Internal Treatments

(1) Toxins Blocking and Stagnation

Zheng: Distension and fullness inside the ear, like being blocked by an external object, hearing loss, tinnitus, lingering for a long time, ear membrane is grey and dipped, blurred, thickened, or has white patches, dizziness, distending pain or sharp pain in the chest, dark tongue with ecchymosis, moderate or hesitant pulse.

Treatment method: Promoting blood circulation, opening up channels, and removing blockages.

Formula: Tong qiao huo xue tang and tong qi san.

(2) Pi Deficiency and Shi Blockage

Zheng: Dull blockage inside the ear, hearing loss, tinnitus with light and dull sound, lingering for a long time. Ear membrane is grey-white and thickened, dipped, or ear membrane is light dark, cloudy, with lack of luster, or is thin and bright. Heavy-headedness and dizziness, fatigue, poor appetite, diarrhea, light swollen tongue, white greasy tai, moderate pulse.

Treatment method: Invigorating the pi and eliminating shi, elevating qing and opening up blockages.

Formula: Bu zhong yi qi tang.

External Treatments

(1) Ear membrane massage: Press and massage the tragus with fingers several dozens times a day.
(2) Pinch the nose and blow to get air into the ear.
(3) Apply di bi ling.

Acupuncture Treatments

(1) Body Acupuncture

Points: Ting gong, ting hui, yi feng, zu san li, pi shu, san yin jiao, shen shu, etc.

(2) Auricular Acupuncture

Points: Er, fei, shen men, shen, pi, shen shang xian, nei fen mi, etc.

Acute Purulent Otitis Media

急 脓 耳

Jí Nóng Ěr

Definition: Acute purulent otitis media is characterized by acute onset of ear pain, pus exuding, and redness, swelling, and perforation of the ear membrane. It happens more frequently in youths and infants. In Chinese medicine, acute purulent otitis media is referred to as ji nong er.

Pathogenesis: Acute purulent otitis media is usually caused by feng heat toxins attacking the ear, gan dan shi heat evaporating upwards, qi and blood getting blocked, and the flesh eroding into pus.

Treatments Based on CM Diagnosis

Internal Treatments

(1) Feng Heat Toxins

Zheng: Acute onset, feeling of dull blockage and pain inside the ear, throbbing pain radiating to the head, hearing loss, ear membrane is bright red and bulging out, some pus exudes, fever, aversion to cold, headache, stuffy nose. For infants, may have crying, morbid night crying, ear-scratching, fever, infantile convulsion, etc. Red tongue tip, thin yellow tai, floating fast pulse.

Treatment method: Clearing heat and detoxifying, driving out feng and relieving the exterior syndrome.

Formula: Wu wei xiao du yin and yin qiao san.

(2) Gan Dan Shi Heat

Zheng: Severe or throbbing pain inside the ear, hearing loss, pus exudes, pain decreases after pus comes out, pus color is yellow and amount is heavy, ear membrane is bright red or dark and bulges out or is perforated, large amount of pus accumulates in the auditory canal, fever, headache, bitter taste, dry throat, constipation, yellow urine, red tongue, yellow greasy tai, stringy fast pulse.

Treatment method: Clearing the gan and dan, detoxifying, and eliminating pus.

Formula: Long dan xie gan tang.

External Treatments

(1) When the ear membrane is red and swollen without perforation, apply ice alcohol drops, three to four times a day.
(2) When pus exudes, clean the pus with 3% hydrogen dioxide solution first. Then apply er yan ling, huang lian di er ye, etc., three to four times a day.
(3) If the ear membrane becomes red, swollen, and bulges out, pus accumulates without exuding, and there is fever and ear pain, perform ear membrane perforation to drain the pus or cut to draw the pus out, clean the pus, and apply er yan ling or huang lian di er ye.

Acupuncture Treatments

Points: Ting gong, ting hui, yi feng, wai guan, yang ling quan, he gu, qu chi.

Chronic Purulent Otitis Media

慢 脓 耳

Màn Nóng Ěr

Definition: Chronic purulent otitis media is characterized by exudates of pus inside the ear and perforation of the ear membrane, which lingers for a long time. In Chinese medicine, chronic purulent otitis media is referred to as man nong er.

Pathogenesis: Chronic purulent otitis media is usually caused by shi heat accumulating inside the ear, eroding the tissues and ear membrane, or pi qi deficiency, shi blocking the auditory canal, shen yin deficiency, and huo of the deficient type burning the ear. If bone tissue is affected, toxins may enter the brain and yin, which is a life-threatening condition.

Treatments Based on CM Diagnosis

Internal Treatments

(1) Shi Heat Accumulation

Zheng: Pus exudes inside the ear, occurs on and off, lingers for a long time, pus color is yellow, thick or thin like water, and may have a foul smell, ear membrane is shi red or dark red with perforation, heavy-headedness, headache, bitter taste, sticky feeling in the mouth, red tongue, yellow greasy tai, soft fast pulse.

Treatment method: Clearing heat and eliminating shi, detoxifying and exuding pus.

Formula: Bi xie shen shi tang.

(2) Pi Deficiency and Shi Blockage

Zheng: Pus exudes inside the ear, occurs on and off, lingers, pus color is white, sticky or dilute, with no foul odor, hearing loss, dizziness, heavy-headedness, perforation of the ear membrane, the edge of the perforation appears white and slightly swollen, fatigue, light swollen tongue, white greasy tai, moderate weak pulse.

Treatment method: Invigorating the pi and nourishing qi, resolving shi and expelling pus.

Formula: Tuo li xiao du san.

(3) Shen Yin Deficiency

Zheng: Pus exudes inside the ear for years, pus is yellow and sticky with a foul odor, or like dirty water, or cheese-like, pus amount is small, ear membrane is perforated severely, the remaining ear membrane appears red and slightly swollen, may affect the bone, dizziness, tinnitus, hearing loss, soreness in the waist and knees, warm sensation in the palms and soles, red tongue, little tai, thin fast pulse.

Treatment method: Nourishing yin and reinforcing the shen, suppressing huo and expelling pus.

Formula: Zhi bo di huang tang.

Acupuncture Treatments

Points: For pi shen deficiency, choose ting gong, ting hui, zu san li, san yin jiao, etc.

11. Rhinology

Nasal Furuncle

鼻 疔

Bí Dīng

Definition: Nasal furuncle is characterized by a small, nail-like furuncle with a firm base around the apex nasi, ala nasi, vestibulum nasi, and may be accompanied by severe pain. In Chinese medicine, nasal furuncle is referred to as bi ding.

Pathogenesis: Nasal furuncle is usually caused by picking the nose, pulling rhinothrix, etc., which cause feng heat toxins to attack the nose, or fei wei heat to accumulate in the nose.

Treatments Based on CM Diagnosis

Internal Treatments

(1) Feng Heat Accumulation

Zheng: Small, rice-like furuncle with a firm base around the external nose or vestibulum nasi, numbness or itchiness, hot sensation, pain, pain intensified by pressing, fever, aversion to cold, discomfort all over the body, light red tongue, thin yellow tai, fast strong pulse.

Treatment method: Driving out feng, clearing heat, detoxifying, and reducing swelling.

Formula: Wu wei xiao du yin.

(2) Excessive Heat Toxins

Zheng: Furuncle around the external nose or vestibulum nasi, tip has a yellow-white pus head, hot and painful sensation, or throbbing pain, swelling may affect the upper lip and area surrounding the nose, fever, headache, discomfort all over the body, constipation, yellow urine, red tongue, yellow tai, fast strong pulse.

Treatment method: Clearing heat, purging huo, reducing swelling, and stopping pain.

Formula: Huang lian jie du tang.

(3) Septicemia Complication

Zheng: Tip of furuncle is dark purple, tip is dipped without pus, base is spread out, nose is swollen like a bottle, severe headache, high fever, vexation, nausea, vomiting, may be accompanied by fainting, delirium, convulsion, tics, red tongue, yellow tai, fast surging pulse.

Treatment method: Purging huo, detoxifying, clearing the ying, and cooling the blood.

Formula: Huang lian jie du tang and xi jiao di huang tang.

Pyogenic Infection of the Nose

鼻 疮

Bí Chuāng

Definition: Pyogenic infection of the nose is characterized by redness, swelling, ulceration with a little pus, hot sensation, itchiness, and pain around the nasal vestibule. In Chinese medicine, pyogenic infection of the nose is referred to as bi chuang.

Pathogenesis: Pyogenic infection of the nose is usually caused by fei channel feng heat, pi wei shi heat, yin and blood deficiency.

Treatments Based on CM Diagnosis

Internal Treatments

(1) Fei Channel Feng Heat

Zheng: Hot sensation, itchiness, pain, redness, swelling, ulceration, yellowish discharge, watery or sticky, scabs, rhagades around the nasal vestibule, warm nasal air, cough with yellow mucus, red tongue tip, thin yellow tai, fast pulse.

Treatment method: Dispersing the fei, clearing heat, driving out feng, and detoxifying.

Formula: Huang qin tang.

(2) Pi Wei Shi Heat

Zheng: Moisture, redness, ulceration around the nasal vestibule, exudes fluid and pus, itchiness, slight pain, thick yellow scabs, lingers for a long time, red tongue, yellow greasy tai, soft fast slippery pulse.

Treatment method: Clearing heat, drying moisture, detoxifying, and regulating the wei.

Formula: Bi xie shen shi tang.

(3) Yin Blood Deficiency

Zheng: Redness, dryness, rhagades, scabs, severe itchiness around the nasal vestibule, a small amount of watery exudates, occurs on and off, drop of vibrissae, skin is rough and thickened, dry mouth and nose, red tongue, little tai, thin fast pulse.

Treatment method: Nourishing yin, supplementing the blood, eliminating dryness, calming down feng.

Formula: Si wu xiao feng yin.

Acute Rhinitis

伤 风 鼻 塞

Shāng Fēng Bí Sāi

Definition: Acute rhinitis is characterized by nasal obstruction, running nose, sneezing, aversion to feng and cold, fever, etc. In Chinese medicine, acute rhinitis is referred to as shang feng bi sai.

Pathogenesis: Acute rhinitis is usually caused by feng cold, feng heat attacks, stagnation in the nose, disturbing the ying and wei.

Treatments Based on CM Diagnosis

Internal Treatments

(1) Feng Cold Attacking the Nose

Zheng: Severely stuffy nose, sneezing frequently, excessive clear nasal discharge, nasal mucosa light red and swollen, headache, aversion to feng and cold, light red tongue, thin white tai, floating tight pulse.

Treatment method: Driving out feng, relieving the exterior syndrome, eliminating cold, and opening up blockages.

Formula: Tong qiao tang.

(2) Feng Heat Attacking the Nose

Zheng: Nasal obstruction on and off, nasal itchiness, warm nasal air, nasal discharge yellow and thick, sneezing frequently, nasal mucosa red or bright red and swollen, fever, mild aversion to feng and cold, thirst, red tongue, thin yellow tai, floating fast pulse.

Treatment method: Driving out feng, relieving the exterior syndrome, clearing heat, opening up blockages.

Formula: Yin qiao san.

Acupuncture Treatments

Points: Ying xiang, yin tang, he gu, tai yang, feng chi.

Chronic Rhinitis

鼻窒

Bí Zhì

Definition: Chronic rhinitis is characterized by chronic nasal obstruction, occurring on and off, or alternative obstruction of both nostrils, or continuous obstruction for a long time, accompanied by decreased osphresis. In Chinese medicine, chronic rhinitis is referred to as bi zhi.

Pathogenesis: Chronic rhinitis is usually caused by fei wei heat attacking the nose, fei pi qi deficiency, cold shi blocking the nose, toxins accumulating in the nose, and qi blood stagnation.

Treatments Based on CM Diagnosis

Internal Treatments

(1) Fei Wei Heat

Zheng: Nasal obstruction on and off for a long time, yellow and thick nasal discharge, hot nasal air, decreased osphresis, headache, red and swollen nasal mucosa and concha, cough with yellow phlegm, red tongue tip, thin yellow tai, shi strong pulse.

Treatment method: Clearing the fei and wei, dispersing stagnation, and opening up blockages.

Formula: Huang qin tang.

(2) Fei Deficiency and Cold Attack

Zheng: Nasal obstruction on and off or alternating obstruction of both nostrils, clear nasal discharge, nasal obstruction gets worse with feng cold, light red and swollen nasal mucosa, swollen and soft concha, weakness, fatigue, cough with white mucus, pale complexion, easily catching cold, light red tongue, white tai, weak pulse.

Treatment method: Reinforcing the fei, nourishing qi, dispersing cold, and opening up blockages.

Formula: Wen fei zhi liu dan.

(3) Pi Deficiency and Shi Blockage

Zheng: Nasal obstruction alternating between nostrils for a long time, excessive nasal discharge, color of mucus is white in general and occasionally yellow, light red, swollen, and soft or slightly hard nasal mucosa and concha, fatigue, poor appetite, diarrhea, heavy-headedness, dizziness, light red tongue with teeth prints, white greasy tai, moderate weak pulse.

Treatment method: Reinforcing the pi, supplementing qi, resolving shi, and opening up blockages.

Formula: Bu zhong yi qi tang.

(4) Qi Blood Stagnation

Zheng: Continuous nasal obstruction which is relieved after movements, excessive thick, white or yellow nasal discharge, decreased or loss of osphresis, nasal sound, dizziness, feeling of swelling in the head, dark red nasal mucosa, swollen and hard concha with a rough surface, dark tongue with ecchymosis, thin hesitant pulse.

Treatment method: Promoting blood circulation, removing stasis, opening channels, and dispersing clots.

Formula: Tong qiao huo xue tang and cang er san.

Acupuncture Treatments

(1) Body Acupuncture

Points: Ying xiang, he gu, shang xing, feng chi, tai yang, yin tang.

(2) Auricular Acupuncture

Points: Bi, nei bi, fei, pi, wei, nei fen mi.

(3) Moxibustion

Points: Ren zhong, ying xiang, feng fu, bai hui.

Acute Nasal Sinusitis

急 鼻 渊

Jí Bí Yuān

Definition: Acute nasal sinusitis is characterized by acute onset with excessive continuous turbid nasal discharge, headache, fever, aversion to cold, discomfort all over the body, and nasal obstruction, etc. In Chinese medicine, acute nasal sinusitis is referred to as ji bi yuan.

Pathogenesis: Acute nasal sinusitis is usually caused by fei channel heat, feng heat, gan dan shi heat, pi wei huo, etc., attacking the sinus.

Treatments Based on CM Diagnosis

Internal Treatments

(1) Fei Channel Feng Heat

Zheng: Sudden turbid nasal discharge as thick as pus, nasal obstruction, decreased osphresis, red and swollen nasal mucosa, swollen concha, pressing pain in the forehead or zygomatic region, headache, fever, aversion to cold, cough, yellow mucus, red tongue tip, thin yellow tai, floating fast pulse.

Treatment method: Clearing heat, dispersing the fei, driving away feng, and opening up blockages.

Formula: Yin qiao san and cang er san.

(2) Gan Dan Shi Heat

Zheng: Excessive turbid foul-smelling nasal discharge, yellowish like pus, nasal obstruction, decreased osphresis, bright red and swollen nasal mucosa, mucus accumulates in the nasal meatus and sinus, headache, pressing pain in the forehead and zygomatic region, fever, bitter taste, dry throat, fast temper, flushing face, conjunctival congestion, tongue red, yellow greasy tai, stringy fast pulse.

Treatment method: Clearing the gan and dan, eliminating shi, and opening up blockages.

Formula: Long dan xie gan tang.

(3) Pi Wei Huo

Zheng: Excessive thick, foul-smelling, pus-like nasal discharge, may be accompanied by clots, nasal obstruction, decreased osphresis, headache especially at the forehead, bright red or dark swollen nasal mucosa, fever, thirst, fondness for cold drinks, foul smell in the mouth, constipation, or swelling pain in the gums, red tongue, yellow tai, surging fast pulse.

Treatment method: Clearing pi and wei, detoxifying, and eliminating mucus.

Formula: Qing wei san.

Acupuncture Treatments

Points: Yin tang, ying xiang, he gu, lie que, tai yang, feng chi, and qu chi, etc.

Chronic Nasal Sinusitis

慢 鼻 渊

Màn Bí Yuān

Definition: Chronic nasal sinusitis is characterized by turbid nasal discharge, occurring on and off for a long time, headache, decreased osphresis, etc. In Chinese medicine, chronic nasal sinusitis is referred to as man bi yuan.

Pathogenesis: Chronic nasal sinusitis is usually caused by fei channel heat attacking the sinus, shi heat blocking the sinus, toxin accumulation, qi blood stasis, gan shen yin deficiency, deficient huo attacking the nose, fei pi qi deficiency, cold shi accumulating in the sinus, etc.

Treatments Based on CM Diagnosis

Internal Treatments

(1) Fei Channel Heat

Zheng: Small amount of foul-smelling turbid nasal discharge, nasal obstruction, decreased osphresis, dizziness, headache, red nasal mucosa, thickened sinus mucosa, warm nasal air, yellow mucus, red tongue tip, thin yellow tai, fast pulse.

Treatment method: Clearing and dispersing fei heat, detoxifying, and removing mucus.

Formula: Huang qin tang.

(2) Shi Heat Blockage

Zheng: Large amount of foul-smelling yellow thick nasal discharge, severe nasal obstruction, heavy-headedness, headache, gets worse in the afternoon, moist, red, and thickened nasal mucosa, polypoid change in the middle concha, lower concha atrophy, thickened sinus mucosa, may be accompanied by mucus accumulation, on and off for a long time, red tongue, yellow greasy tai, soft fast pulse.

Treatment method: Clearing heat, resolving shi, eliminating blockages, and removing mucus.

Formula: Juan bi tong qiao tang.

(3) Qi Blood Stagnation

Zheng: White or yellow thick nasal discharge, headache without fixed time, dark red and thickened nasal mucosa, thickened sinus mucosa, dark tongue with ecchymosis, thin hesitant pulse.

Treatment method: Promoting blood circulation, removing qi stagnation, and dispersing blockages.

Formula: Tong qiao huo xue tang and cang er san.

(4) Gan Shen Yin Deficiency

Zheng: Small amount of turbid nasal discharge, decreased osphresis, headache with deficient feeling around the vertex and occiput, or continuous dull headache, dizziness, tinnitus, amnesia, hot palms and soles, soreness and weakness in the waist and knees, slightly red and swollen nasal mucosa, lower concha atrophy, sinus mucosa thickening or atrophy, slight osteoporosis, red tongue, little tai, thin fast pulse.

Treatment method: Nourishing the gan and shen, eliminating huo, and removing mucus.

Formula: Qi ju di huang tang.

(5) Fei Pi Qi Deficiency

Zheng: White or clear nasal discharge without foul smell, amount fluctuates, nasal obstruction, decreased osphresis, dizziness, heavy-headedness, headache with cool feeling, slightly red or dark nasal mucosa, thickened sinus mucosa, polypoid change in the middle concha, fatigue, weakness, low voice, spontaneous perspiration, aversion to feng, easily catching cold, poor appetite, diarrhea, pale complexion, spitting white mucus, condition gets worse with feng cold or exertion, light red tongue, white tai, moderate weak pulse.

Treatment method: Reinforcing the pi and fei, dispersing cold, and resolving shi.

Formula: Shen ling bai zhu san.

Acupuncture Treatments

(1) Body Acupuncture

Points: Ying xiang, he gu, yin tang, tai yang, feng chi, zu san li, etc.

(2) Auricular Acupuncture

Points: Nei bi, e, fei, wei, pi, shen, nei fen mi, etc.

Nasopharyngeal Carcinoma

鼻 咽 癌

Bí Yān Ái

Definition: Nasopharyngeal carcinoma may not show any symptoms in the early stage. As it progresses, it is characterized by blood in nasal discharge, nosebleed, tinnitus, loss of hearing, stuffy ear, stuffy nose, headache, enlarged lymph nodes, vision disturbances, etc. In Chinese medicine, nasopharyngeal carcinoma is referred to as bi zhi, shi rong, etc.

Pathogenesis: Nasopharyngeal carcinoma is usually caused by fei heat toxins, gan qi stagnation, tan huo attack, etc.

Treatments Based on CM Diagnosis

Internal Treatments

(1) Gan Fei Stagnant Heat

Zheng: Stuffy nose, blood in nasal discharge, nosebleed, cough, little sticky phlegm, bitter taste, dry throat, vexation, fast temper, dizziness, headache, red tongue, yellow tai, stringy slippery fast pulse.

Treatment method: Clearing the gan and purging the fei.

Formula: Dan zhi xiao yao san.

(2) Tan Heat Accumulation

Zheng: Stuffy nose, turbid nasal discharge, blood in nasal discharge, enlarged neck lymph nodes, and may be accompanied by facial hemiparalysis, headache, dark tongue, thick greasy tai, stringy slippery fast pulse.

Treatment method: Dissolving tan and resolving stagnation, clearing heat and detoxifying.

Formula: Qing jin hua tan tang.

(3) Fei Shen Yin Deficiency

Zheng: Dizziness, tinnitus, deafness, blurred vision, hoarse voice, soreness in the waist and knees, tidal heat, night sweats, red tongue, little tai or thin yellow tai, thin fast weak pulse.

Treatment method: Nourishing the fei and shen.

Formula: Mai wei di huang tang.

12. Laryngology

Acute Tonsillitis

急 乳 蛾

Jí Rǔ É

Definition: Acute tonsillitis is characterized by acute onset of pain, hotness, redness of the throat, pharyngeal tonsil swollen or ulcerated, jeopardizing the swallowing process, fever, whole body discomfort, etc. In Chinese medicine, acute tonsillitis is referred to as ji ru e.

Pathogenesis: Acute tonsillitis is usually caused by fei channel heat, combined with feng heat and fei wei heat, attacking the throat, blocking qi and the blood.

Treatments Based on CM Diagnosis

Internal Treatments

(1) Fei Channel Feng Heat

Zheng: Acute onset of dry pain and hot throat, difficulty swallowing, red and swollen throat, swollen pharyngeal tonsil, fever, aversion to cold, red tongue tip, thin yellow tai, floating fast pulse.

Treatment method: Driving out feng, clearing heat, detoxifying, and soothing the throat.

Formula: Shu feng qing re tang.

(2) Fei Wei Excessive Heat

Zheng: Severe sore throat, pain radiating to the ears, difficulty swallowing, red and swollen throat, bright red and swollen pharyngeal tonsil with yellow-whitish pus and ulceration, or pseudomembrane, submaxillary pressing pain, high fever, flushed face, thirst, foul-smelling mouth, constipation, red tongue, yellow tai, strong fast pulse.

Treatment method: Purging the fei and wei, detoxifying, and soothing the throat.

Formula: Qing yan li ge tang.

Acupuncture Treatments

Points: He gu, nei ting, qu chi, tian tu, shao ze, yu ji, etc.

Chronic Tonsillitis

慢　乳　蛾

Màn　Rŭ　É

Definition: Chronic tonsillitis is characterized by an enlarged red or dark red tonsil, uneven tonsil surface, having yellow-white pus spots, lingering for a long time, repeated relapses, feeling of discomfort in the throat, feeling of a foreign body located in the throat, foul-smelling mouth, exuding a yellow-whitish discharge when pressing the front of the throat, or a shrunken tonsil attached to the anterior and posterior walls of the throat. In Chinese medicine, chronic tonsillitis is referred to as man ru e.

Pathogenesis: Chronic tonsillitis is usually caused by delayed or inappropriate treatment of acute tonsillitis, toxins accumulating in the tonsil, fei shen yin deficiency, fei pi qi deficiency, and qi blood stasis, etc.

Treatments Based on CM Diagnosis

Internal Treatments

(1) Fei Shen Yin Deficiency

Zheng: Dryness, itchiness, and slight pain in the throat, difficulty swallowing, worsens in the afternoon and evening, red or dark red isthmus of the fauces and tonsil, enlarged soft tonsil, exuding small amounts of decayed tissue when pressed, dry cough with little mucus, tidal fever in the afternoon, hot palms and soles, soreness in the waist and knees, red tongue, little tai, thin fast pulse.

Treatment method: Nourishing the fei and shen, quenching huo, and eliminating inflammation.

Formula: Bai he gu jin tang.

(2) Fei Pi Qi Deficiency

Zheng: Slightly dry throat, feeling of discomfort similar to that of having a foreign body in the throat, slightly red or dark enlarged soft tonsil, fluctuating amount of exudates of white pus without foul smell, lingering for a long time, fatigue, no taste in the mouth, no dry mouth or thirst, easily catching cold, poor appetite, diarrhea, light red tongue, white tai, moderate weak pulse.

Treatment method: Reinforcing the pi and fei, resolving shi, and removing inflammation.

Formula: Bu zhong yi qi tang.

(3) Qi Blood Blockage

Zheng: Dry throat, difficulty swallowing, feeling of discomfort similar to that of having a foreign body blocking the throat, stabbing or distending pain, on and off, dark red isthmus of the fauces, enlarged hard tonsil with uneven surface, tonsil enlargement lingers for a long time, dark tongue with ecchymosis, deep hesitant pulse.

Treatment method: Promoting blood circulation, dispersing blockages, and removing inflammation.

Formula: Huo xue li yan tang.

Acupuncture Treatments

(1) Body Acupuncture

Points: He gu, qu chi, zu san li, jia che, tian rong, san yin jiao, fei shu, pi shu, shen shu, etc.

(2) Auricular Acupuncture

Points: Bian tao ti, yan, fei, shen, pi, nei fen mi, etc.

Acute Pharyngitis

急 喉 痹

Jí Hóu Bì

Definition: Acute pharyngitis is characterized by acute onset of redness, swelling, pain, dryness, hotness, itchiness around the pharynx, pain increases during swallowing, pain may radiate to the ear, fever, headache, cough, whole body discomfort, red nodules at the bottom of the larynx, thick yellow mucus, red and swollen retropharyngeal column and uvula. In Chinese medicine, acute pharyngitis is referred to as ji hou bi.

Pathogenesis: Acute pharyngitis is usually caused by feng cold attacking the pharynx, fei channel heat, external feng heat, and fei wei tan heat accumulating in the pharynx.

Treatments Based on CM Diagnosis

Internal Treatments

(1) Feng Cold Attack

Zheng: Sudden feeling of discomfort, swelling, pain, itchiness of the pharynx, light white red and slightly swollen pharyngeal cavity myolemma, aversion to cold, mild fever, headache, heavy limbs, cough, dilute mucus, no thirst, light red tongue, thin white tai, floating tight pulse.

Treatment method: Driving out feng, clearing cold, dispersing the lung, and soothing the pharynx.

Formula: Liu wei tang.

(2) Fei Channel Feng Heat

Zheng: Acute onset of dryness, hotness, and pain in the pharynx, progressively worsens, red and swollen pharyngeal cavity, retropharyngeal column, and uvula, red nodules at the the bottom of the larynx, fever, aversion to cold, cough, yellow mucus, red tongue tip, thin yellow tai, floating fast pulse.

Treatment method: Driving out feng, clearing heat, detoxifying, and relieving the pharynx.

Formula: Shu feng qing re tang.

(3) Fei Wei Tan Heat

Zheng: Dryness, hotness, and severe pain in the pharynx, pain increases during swallowing, red and swollen pharyngeal cavity, plenty of red nodules at the bottom of the larynx covered with yellow-white mucus, tonsil may become red and swollen, swelling and pain in the submaxillary gland, fever, headache, cough, large amounts of yellow thick mucus, thirst, constipation, red tongue, yellow greasy tai, slippery fast surging pulse.

Treatment method: Clearing heat, purging huo, resolving phlegm, and relieving the pharynx.

Formula: Qing re li yan tang.

Acupuncture Treatments

Points: He gu, nei ting, qu chi, shao ze, shao shang, shang yang, etc.

Chronic Pharyngitis

慢　喉　痹

Màn Hóu Bì

Definition: Chronic pharyngitis is characterized by dryness, red or dark red or white color, discomfort, pain, itchiness, hotness, and swelling around the pharynx, feeling of having a foreign object in the throat, small nodules at the bottom of the larynx, difficulty swallowing, lingering for a long time. In Chinese medicine, chronic pharyngitis is referred to as man hou bi.

Pathogenesis: Chronic pharyngitis is usually caused by fei shen yin deficiency, gan channel stagnant heat, qi blood stagnation, tan shi accumulation, and shen yang deficiency.

Treatments Based on CM Diagnosis

Internal Treatments

(1) Fei Shen Yin Deficiency

Zheng: Dryness, itchiness, slight pain, and hot sensation in the pharynx, worsens at night, slightly red and swollen pharyngeal cavity, thirst, some red nodules at the the bottom of the larynx, dry cough, little mucus, soreness in the waist and knees, hot palms and soles, red tongue, little tai, thin fast pulse.

Treatment method: Nourishing the fei and shen, reducing huo and relieving the pharynx.

Formula: Bai he gu jin tang.

(2) Gan Channel Stagnant Heat

Zheng: Feeling of discomfort and blockage in the pharynx, prominent feeling of foreign object obstruction, worsens with undesired emotions, red or dark red pharyngeal cavity, many red nodules at the bottom of the larynx, fast temper, chest and hypochondriac distension, bitter taste, red tongue edge, yellow tai, stringy fast pulse.

Treatment method: Soothing the gan and clearing heat, regulating qi and relieving the pharynx.

Formula: Dan zhi xiao yao san.

(3) Qi Blood Stagnation

Zheng: Dryness, itchiness, hot sensation, and distending pain in the pharynx, difficulty swallowing, worsens at night, relieved after movement, dark red and thickened pharyngeal cavity, small nodules at the bottom of the larynx, dark tongue with ecchymosis, white or yellow tai, thin hesitant pulse.

Treatment method: Promoting blood circulation, regulating qi, and relieving the pharynx.

Formula: Huo xue li yan tang.

(4) Tan Shi Accumulation

Zheng: Feeling of discomfort in the pharynx, difficulty swallowing, prominent feeling of tan blockage, white or slightly red pharyngeal cavity, many small nodules at the bottom of the larynx covered with white mucus, chest and hypochondriac distension, nausea, poor appetite, sticky mouth, plenty of white mucus, light tongue, white greasy tai, stringy slippery pulse.

Treatment method: Eliminating shi and resolving phlegm, dispersing blockages and relieving the pharynx.

Formula: Dao tan tang.

(5) Shen Yang Deficiency

Zheng: Feeling of discomfort and blockage around the pharynx, light white and swollen or dark thickened pharyngeal cavity, no thirst, tastelessness, relieved by drinking hot water, pale complexion, cold limbs, soreness in the waist and back, fatigue, light red tongue, white tai, deep weak pulse.

Treatment method: Warming the shen and strengthening yang, clearing cold and relieving the pharynx.

Formula: Jin gui shen qi wan.

Acupuncture Treatments

Points: He gu, tian tu, fu tu, lian quan, san yin jiao, etc.

Acute Laryngitis

急　喉　瘖

Jí　Hóu　Yīn

Definition: Acute laryngitis is characterized by acute onset of hoarseness, aphonia, red and swollen laryngeal myolemma, dry, hot, and painful sensation, cough, red and swollen larynx and vocal cord with sticky exudates. In Chinese medicine, acute laryngitis is referred to as ji hou yin.

Pathogenesis: Acute laryngitis is usually caused by fei channel heat, feng heat, feng cold, or fei wei tan heat attacking the laryngx.

Treatments Based on CM Diagnosis

Internal Treatments

(1) Feng Cold Attacking the Larynx

Zheng: Sudden loss of voice or hoarseness, light pain and itchiness of the larynx, slightly white or red and swollen laryngeal myolemma, slightly red vocal cord, frequent coughing, stuffy nose, clear nasal discharge, aversion to cold, fever, headache, no sweating, red tongue, thin white tai, floating tight pulse.

Treatment method: Driving out feng and clearing cold, dispersing the lung and restoring voice.

Formula: Liu wei tang.

(2) Fei Channel Feng Heat

Zheng: Hoarse voice or loss of voice, hot, dry, itchy, and painful feeling in the larynx, pain increases during coughing, red and swollen laryngeal myolemma, vocal cord is red and cannot close properly, fever, aversion to feng, thirst, red tongue tip, thin yellow tai, floating fast pulse.

Treatment method: Driving out feng and clearing heat, dispersing the lung and restoring voice.

Formula: Sang ju yin.

(3) Fei Wei Tan Heat

Zheng: Hoarseness, hot and painful larynx, worsens when coughing and speaking, yellow and thick mucus, bright red and swollen laryngeal myolemma and vocal cord with mucus, thirst, bitter taste, poor appetite, constipation, fever, red tongue, yellow greasy tai, fast pulse.

Treatment method: Clearing the fei and wei, resolving tan and restoring voice.

Formula: Qing re li yan tang.

Acupuncture Treatments

Points: He gu, qu chi, tian tu, da zhui, ren ying, etc.

Chronic Laryngitis

慢 喉 瘖

Màn Hóu Yīn

Definition: Chronic laryngitis is characterized by hoarseness or loss of voice, thickened, red, dull and swollen laryngeal myolemma or vocal cord, lingering for a long time, fluctuating, worsening when speaking frequently, hot, dry, and itchy feeling in the larynx, feeling of blockage by a foreign object, dry cough, little mucus, expanded vessels in the larynx, failure of the glottis to close properly. In Chinese medicine, chronic laryngitis is referred to as man hou yin.

Pathogenesis: Chronic laryngitis is usually caused by delayed or failed treatment of acute laryngitis, lack of maintenance, toxin attack, fei pi shen qi and yin deficiency, qi and blood blockage, etc.

Treatments Based on CM Diagnosis

Internal Treatments

(1) Fei Shen Yin Deficiency

Zheng: Loss of voice or hoarseness, lingering for a long time, worsening when speaking frequently and in the afternoon, recovering in the early morning, dry, hot, itchy, and slightly painful larynx, dry cough, little mucus, slightly red and swollen, dull and dry laryngeal myolemma and vocal cord, failure of the glottis to close properly, hot palms and soles, soreness in the waist and knees, red tongue, little tai, thin fast pulse.

Treatment method: Nourishing the fei and shen, eliminating huo and soothing the larynx.

385

Formula: Bai he gu jin tang.

(2) Fei Pi Qi Deficiency

Zheng: Loss of voice or hoarseness, lingering for a long time, worsening in the morning or after exertion, light white, red or dark laryngeal myolemma or vocal cord, vocal cord is thickened and cannot close properly, fatigue, shortness of breath, spontaneous perspiration, poor appetite, diarrhea, light red tongue, white tai, moderate weak pulse.

Treatment method: Reinforcing the pi and nourishing the fei, ascending qing and resolving shi.

Formula: Bu zhong yi qi tang and he zi yin.

(3) Tan Blood Stasis

Zheng: Hoarseness for a long time, swollen, rough larynx with stabbing pain, feeling of foreign object obstruction, laryngeal myolemma or vocal cord dark is red and thickened and cannot close properly, white thick mucus, dark tongue with ecchymosis, greasy tai, hesitant or moderate pulse.

Treatment method: Promoting blood circulation and removing stasis, resolving tan and dispersing blockages.

Formula: Hui yan zhu yu tang and er chen tang.

Acupuncture Treatments

Points: Tian tu, lian quan, ren ying, zu san li, san yin jiao, fei shu, shen shu, pi shu, etc.

13. Stomatology

Toothache

牙 痛

Yá Tòng

Definition: Toothache is characterized by tooth pain, on and off, or lasting for a long time, and may be accompanied by red and swollen gums. It is often a symptom of many tooth diseases and periodontal diseases. In Chinese medicine, toothache is referred to as ya tong.

Pathogenesis: Toothache is usually caused by feng cold, feng huo, wei huo, and deficient huo attacking the tooth.

Treatments Based on CM Diagnosis

Internal Treatments

(1) Feng Cold Toothache

Zheng: Toothache, relieved by warmth and worsens with coldness, tastelessness, no thirst, slightly white or red gums, light red tongue, thin white tai, floating tight pulse.

Treatment method: Driving out feng, dispersing cold, and stopping pain.

Formula: Ma huang fu zi xi xin tang.

(2) Feng Huo Toothache

Zheng: Toothache occurs on and off, relieved by cold, worsens with heat, fever, aversion to cold, thirst, constipation, red tongue tip, thin yellow tai, floating fast pulse.

Treatment method: Driving out feng, clearing huo, and stopping pain.

Formula: Fang feng tong sheng san.

(3) Wei Huo Toothache

Zheng: Severe continuous toothache, secreting warm saliva, red and swollen gums, may be accompanied by parotid gland swelling, thirst, halitosis, constipation, red tongue, yellow tai, surging fast pulse.

Treatment method: Clearing the stomach and purging huo, cooling the blood and stopping pain.

Formula: Qing wei san.

(4) Deficient Huo Toothache

Zheng: Dull toothache occurs on and off and lasts for a long time, slightly red and swollen gums, loose teeth, lacking strength in bite, soreness in the waist and knees, dizziness, tinnitus, hot palms and soles, red tongue, little tai, thin fast pulse.

Treatment method: Nourishing yin and clearing huo, strengthening the shen and reinforcing teeth.

Formula: Zhi bo di huang san.

Acupuncture Treatments

Points for upper toothache: Xia guan, nei ting, he gu.
Points for lower toothache: Jia che, he gu.
Additional points for feng huo toothache: Tai yang, feng chi.
Additional points for wei huo toothache: Quan liao, zu san li.
Additional points for deficient huo toothache: Tai xi, san yin jiao.

Gingival Abscess

牙 痈

Yá Yōng

Definition: Gingival abscess is characterized by localized red swelling and abscess of the gums with severe pain. In Chinese medicine, gingival abscess is referred to as ya yong.

Pathogenesis: Gingival abscess is usually caused by pi wei heat and feng heat eroding the gingival tissues and forming abscess.

Treatments Based on CM Diagnosis

Internal Treatment

Zheng: At the beginning, the gums become red, swollen, and hard, with burning sensation and pain, symptoms decrease with coldness and increase during mastication, abscess gradually forms, constant throbbing pain, pain decreases after pus exudes, may affect the parotid cheek and mandible, pressing pain in the submaxillary gland, fever, headache, halitosis, constipation, red tongue, yellow tai, surging fast pulse.

Treatment method: Clearing heat and purging huo, eliminating swelling and stopping pain.

Formula: Qing wei san and wu wei xiao du yin.

Acupuncture Treatments

Points: He gu, jia che, xia guan, etc.

Gingival Atrophy

牙 宣

Yá Xuān

Definition: Gingival atrophy is characterized by gingival ulceration and atrophy, exposure of the root of the tooth, loose teeth, exuding blood and pus. In Chinese medicine, gingival atrophy is referred to as ya xuan.

Pathogenesis: Gingival atrophy is usually caused by wei huo flaming up, shen yin deficiency, and qi blood deficiency.

Treatments Based on CM Diagnosis

Internal Treatments

(1) Wei Huo Flaming Up

Zheng: Red, swollen, painful, and ulcerated gums, exuding large amounts of foul-smelling blood and pus, odontolith accumulates, gum atrophy, hunger, constipation, red tongue, yellow tai, surging fast pulse.

Treatment method: Clearing the wei and purging huo, detoxifying and eliminating swelling.

Formula: Qing wei san.

(2) Shen Yin Deficiency

Zheng: Gum atrophy, ulceration, root of tooth exposed, red and swollen gums, exuding blood, loose teeth, mild pain, lingering for a long time, progressing gradually, dizziness, tinnitus, soreness in the waist and knees, red tongue, little tai, thin fast pulse.

Treatment method: Nourishing the shen and reinforcing jing, nurturing the gums and strengthening teeth.

Formula: Liu wei di huang tang.

(3) Qi Blood Deficiency

Zheng: Light white gums, gum atrophy, root of tooth exposed, loose teeth, lacking strength in mastication, exuding small amount of light red blood, lingering for a long time, pale complexion, fatigue, light red tongue, white tai, weak pulse.

Treatment method: Nourishing qi and nurturing the blood, reinforcing the gums and strengthening teeth.

Formula: Ba zhen tang.

Acupuncture Treatments

Points: He gu, nei ting, jia che, xia guan, zu san li, san yin jiao, etc.

Aphthae

口　疮

Kǒu Chuāng

Definition: Aphthae is characterized by shallow ulceration of the mouth cavity myolemma, commonly seen in youths. In Chinese medicine, aphthae is referred to as kou chuang.

Pathogenesis: Aphthae is usually caused by xin pi heat, yin deficiency and huo flaming up, and pi wei deficiency, etc.

Treatments Based on CM Diagnosis

Internal Treatments

(1) Xin Pi Heat

Zheng: Mouth cavity myolemma ulceration, ulcerating surface is yellow, dipping in the middle, surrounding myolemma is bright red and swollen, multiple aphthae which may merge together, hot sensation, pain, fever, bitter taste, halitosis, thirst, fondness for cold drinks, constipation, yellow urine, red tongue, yellow tai, fast pulse.

Treatment method: Clearing the xin and cooling the pi, eliminating swelling and stopping pain.

Formula: Liang ge san.

(2) Yin Deficiency and Huo Flaming Up

Zheng: Mouth cavity myolemma ulceration, ulcerating surface is pale and yellow, surrounding area is slightly red and swollen, mild pain, on and off for a long time, dry mouth, vexation, insomnia, soreness in the waist and knees, hot palms and soles, red tongue, little tai, thin fast pulse.

Treatment method: Nourishing the xin and shen, eliminating huo and reducing aphthae.

Formula: Zhi bo di huang tang or tian wang bu xin dan.

(3) Pi Wei Deficiency

Zheng: Mouth cavity myolemma ulceration, on and off repeatedly for a long time, ulceration surface is pale, surrounding area is dark and slightly swollen, no redness, no pain or mild pain, fatigue, poor appetite, diarrhea, light red tongue, white tai, moderate weak pulse.

Treatment method: Reinforcing the pi and nourishing qi, ascending qing and resolving shi.

Formula: Bu zhong yi qi tang.

Acupuncture Treatments

Points: Lian quan, zu san li, he gu, qu chi, jia che, di cang, san yin jiao, etc.

Fissured Tongue

舌 裂

Shé Liè

Definition: Fissured tongue is characterized by fissure(s) on the lingual surface without other symptoms. Sometimes it is accompanied by dry mouth, stabbing pain, itchiness, etc. In Chinese medicine, fissured tongue is referred to as she lie.

Pathogenesis: Fissured tongue is usually caused by xin channel heat, xin pi yin deficiency, gan shen yin deficiency, etc.

Treatments Based on CM Diagnosis

Internal Treatments

(1) Xin Channel Heat

Zheng: Red or bright red tongue with fissures on the surface, may be accompanied by swelling, especially at the tip of the tongue, hotness, dryness, pain, vexation, insomnia, bitter taste, halitosis, yellow urine, fast pulse.

Treatment method: Clearing the xin and purging heat, cooling the blood and eliminating swelling.

Formula: Dao chi san and xi jiao di huang tang.

(2) Xin Pi Yin Deficiency

Zheng: Red tongue, dry and fissured surface, itchy with mild pain or no pain, lingering for a long time, vexation, insomnia, excessive dreaming, anorexia, thin fast pulse.

Treatment method: Nourishing the xin and pi, clearing heat and reinforcing yin.

Formula: Yi wei tang.

(3) Gan Shen Yin Deficiency

Zheng: Light red tongue, dry and fissured surface, fissures similar to ditches especially in the posterior part, atrophy, hotness, mild pain, lingering for a long time, dizziness, tinnitus, soreness in the waist and knees, hot palms and soles, thin fast pulse.

Treatment method: Nourishing the gan and shen, clearing deficient huo.

Formula: Qi ju di huang tang.

14. Preventive Medicine

In the preceding chapters we have mainly focused on disease treatments. However, if a disease can be prevented, further treatments will be avoided. Due to this reason, *Nei Jing* states: "A sage treats a disease before the disease occurs, and governs a disorder before the disorder starts." As a result, disease prevention has become the foremost task in Chinese medicine, and preventive medicine has become a very important component in Chinese medicine.

Chinese preventive medicine can be divided into two categories: preventing disease from occurring and preventing disease from developing.

Preventing Disease from Occurring

Preventing disease from occurring involves taking measures before the advent of disease. Concretely speaking, Chinese medicine employs the following measures to prevent a disease from occurring.

Reinforcing Zheng Qi

Su Wen states: "With zheng qi inside, xie qi is unable to get in." In Chinese medicine, zheng qi is a sum of all factors contributing to improving the body's immune system and recovery capability. Xie qi refers to all pathogenic factors and pathological damage capable of causing diseases and illnesses. Therefore, by reinforcing zheng qi, xie qi cannot attack the body and disease can be prevented. Specifically, the ways to reinforce zheng qi are as follows:

(1) Regulating the Mind and Spirit

In Chinese medicine, the mind and spirit have very important relationships with physiological and pathological conditions of the human body. The mind and spirit can directly cause illnesses. They can also indirectly introduce diseases by lowering the body's zheng qi.

Therefore, by regulating the mind and spirit, one can reinforce zheng qi, improve the immune function, and prevent disease from occurring or developing, and can help the body recover from existing illnesses.

(2) Exercise

According to Chinese medicine, life is rooted in movement. Based on this principle, Chinese medicine has developed wu qin xi, tai ji, ba duan jin, qi gong, dao yin, and many other forms of therapeutic exercise.

Frequent exercise can improve the body's zheng qi, improve the immune function, prevent disease from occurring or developing, and can help the body to recover from existing illnesses.

(3) Regulating Lifestyle

Chinese medicine stresses the importance of a healthy lifestyle in the prevention of diseases. With respect to diet, Chinese medicine emphasizes a balanced diet with appropriate quantity and quality.

In daily life, regularity is highly recommended. It is important to adjust the schedule according to the seasons. Work, rest, and recreation should be alternated to reach a balance in order to prevent illnesses and to prolong the life span.

(4) Immunology

The world's first vaccination technique was developed in Chinese medicine hundreds of years ago. Artificial immunization can enhance the body's zheng qi, improve the immune function, and help prevent diseases.

Eliminating Xie Qi

Xie qi is an important factor leading to diseases. Therefore, in addition to reinforcing zheng qi, eliminating xie qi is also very important in preventing diseases. Specifically, the ways to eliminating xie qi are as follows:

(1) Removing Xie Qi by Herbal Medicine

The following methods are used in removing xie qi in Chinese herbal medicine:

(i)   Burning and fumigating: This method involves burning and fumigating appropriate herbs in order to destroy xie qi. It is used to remove xie qi in the environment, room, etc.

(ii) Wearing: This method involves wearing herbal medicine bags in order to drive xie qi away. The herbal bag usually is hung in front of the chest, no more than 10 cm from the nose. It is used to prevent cold, flu, poor appetite, and nasal diseases.

(iii) Bathing: This method involves letting the patient sit in a bathtub filled with a decoction of herbal medicine. It is used to prevent many diseases by removing xie qi from the skin of the body.

(iv) Topical application: This method involves applying herbal cream, lotion, etc., to certain areas of the skin in order to remove xie qi and prevent many diseases.

(v)   Oral administration: This method involves letting the patient take herbs orally in order to remove xie qi from the body and prevent diseases. This is one of the most widely used methods in Chinese medicine.

(2) Hygiene

This includes the following two aspects:

(i)   Food hygiene: It includes food pollution prevention, food quality assurance, poisoning prevention, etc.

(ii) Environmental hygiene: This includes air pollution prevention, ventilation, moisture prevention, house cleaning, waste control, water quality control, etc.

(3) Avoiding Attack of Xie Qi

Avoiding the attack of xie qi includes the following methods:

(i)   Adjusting to weather changes: Chinese medicine emphasizes that people should adjust their lifestyles and clothes so that they are consistent with the weather changes. In this way, xie qi will not have the chance to attack the body. Disregarding weather changes can provide opportunities for xie qi to attack the body.

(ii) Quarantine: For certain epidemic diseases, Chinese medicine recommends taking quarantine measures in order to prevent them from spreading.

(iii) Destroying xie qi: This includes destroying xie qi in the house, on clothes of patients, cleaning wounds, etc.

(4) Avoiding Injury

Weapon wounds, injuries from falls, fractures, contusions, strains, bite wounds from insects and animals, etc., all are pathogenic factors. They fall into the general category of xie qi, and should be avoided.

Preventing Disease from Developing

Preventing disease from occurring in the first place is the ideal in Chinese medicine. However, due to many reasons, this cannot always be achieved. Once a disease has happened, the next preventive measure in Chinese medicine is to prevent it from developing further.

Early Diagnosis and Treatment

Su Wen states: "The arrival of xie qi is similar to a rainstorm. The best treatment begins while the disease is still at the skin level. Secondary treatment starts when the disease propagates to the muscular level. The next treatment targets the tendon and vessel levels. The following treatment concentrates on the six fu organs. The last resort focuses on the five zang organs. The success rate for treating the five zang organs is only about fifty percent." This indicates that the earlier the treatments start, the better the therapeutic outcomes.

Generally speaking, a disease is not serious in the earlier stages. Therefore, appropriate treatments at earlier stages usually can effectively control the disease from developing further and even cure it.

Preventing the Development and Propagation of Diseases

Nan Jing states: "The best doctor treats the non-affected organs, while the ordinary doctor treats the affected organs." This means that the best treatment should focus on the organs that have not been affected yet in order to prevent diseases from propagating to them.

All diseases have their own characteristics and follow certain rules in developing and propagating. Chinese medicine has accumulated many theories describing these rules. For example, exopathic diseases follow six-channel propagation, wei qi yin xue propagation, tri-jiao propagation, etc. Internal injury diseases follow five-zang-organ propagation, zang-fu organ propagation, meridian channel propagation, etc.

Therefore, understanding the disease propagation regularities and taking measures to cut off the disease's developing and propagating pathway can effectively treat and control the disease that already has come into existence.

Appendix I
Acupuncture Points

The following acupuncture points are measured based on the unit cun (寸, cùn). In Chinese medicine, cun is a relative term. Its length varies from patient to patient depending on the patient's body size. For simplicity, a cun is approximately equal to the width of the patient's thumb joint.

Lung Meridian of Hand Tai Yin (LU)

Point locations:

LU1 Zhong fu: 6 cun lateral to the anterior midline level with the first intercostal space, 1 cun below LU2. Caution: needle oblique to avoid lungs.

LU2 Yun men: 6 cun lateral to the anterior midline below the clavicle in the depression medial to the coracoid process. Caution: needle oblique to avoid lungs.

LU3 Tian fu: 3 cun inferior to the anterior axillary fold on the radial side of the biceps brachii muscle.

LU4 Xia bai: 4 cun inferior to the anterior axillary fold, 1 cun inferior to LU3 on the radial side of the biceps brachii muscle.

LU5 Chi ze: On the cubital crease, in the depression lateral to the biceps brachii tendon.

LU6 Kong zui: 7 cun above the transverse crease of the wrist.

LU7 Lie que: 1.5 cun above the transverse crease of the wrist, superior to the styloid process of the radius.

LU8 Jing qu: 1 cun above the transverse crease of the wrist in the hollow on the lateral side of the radial artery.

LU9 Tai yuan: On the transverse crease of the wrist on the lateral side of the radial artery.

LU10 Yu ji: On the palmar side of the hand, at the midpoint of the first metacarpal bone, at the junction of the red and white skin.

LU11 Shao shang: 0.1 cun posterior to the nail on the radial side of the nail.

Large Intestine Meridian of Hand Yang Ming (LI)

Point locations:

LI1 Shang yang: 0.1 cun posterior to the corner of the nail on the radial side of the index finger.

LI2 Er jian: On the radial side of the index finger distal to the second metacarpalphalangeal joint in the depression at the junction of the red and white skin.

LI3 San jian: On the radial side of the index finger proximal to the head of the second metacarpal bone.

LI4 He gu: On the dorsum of the hand, between the first and second metacarpal bones.

LI5 Yang xi: On the radial side of the wrist between the extensor pollicis longus and brevis tendons in a depression formed when the thumb is tilted upward (anatomical snuffbox).

LI6 Pian li: 3 cun above the transverse crease of the wrist (LI5) on the radial side of the forearm.

LI7 Wen liu: 5 cun above the transverse crease of the wrist (LI5) on the radial side of the forearm.

LI8 Xia lian: 4 cun below LI11 on the radial side of the forearm on the line connecting LI5 and LI11.

LI9 Shang lian: 3 cun below LI11 on the radial side of the forearm on the line connecting LI5 and LI11.

LI10 Shou san li: 2 cun below LI11 on the radial side of the forearm on the line connecting LI5 and LI11.

LI11 Qu chi: With a bent elbow, the point lies in the depression at the lateral end of the transverse cubital crease, midway between LU5 and the lateral epicondyle of the humerus.

LI12 Zhou liao: With the elbow flexed, on the radial side of the upper arm 1 cun above and lateral to LI11 on the lateral/posterior border of the humerus.

LI13 Shou wu li: 3 cun above LI11 on the line connecting LI11 and LI15. Avoid injuring the artery when needling.

LI14 Bi nao: 4 cun above LI13 at the inferior border of the deltoid, on the line connecting LI11 and LI15.

LI15 Jian yu: Anterior and inferior to the acromion, on the upper portion of the deltoid muscle, in a depression formed when the arm is in full abduction.

LI16 Ju gu: Slightly posterior to the shoulder, in the depression between the acromion process and the scapular spine.

LI17 Tian ding: On the lateral side of the neck, 1 cun below LI18 on the posterior border of the sternocleidomastoid muscle (SCM).

LI18 Fu tu: On the lateral side of the neck, level with the tip of the Adam's apple between the sternal head and the clavicular head of the SCM.

LI19 Kou he liao: Directly below the lateral margin of the nostril 0.5 cun lateral to DU26.

LI20 Ying xiang: In the nasolabial sulcus, level with the midpoint of the lateral border of the ala nasi.

Stomach Meridian of Foot Yang Ming (ST)

Point locations:

ST1 Cheng qi: Directly below the pupil between the eyeball and the infraorbital ridge.

ST2 Si bai: Directly below the pupil in a depression at the infraorbital foramen.

ST3 Ju liao: Directly below the pupil in a depression level with the lower border of the ala nasi.

ST4 Di cang: Directly below the pupil lateral to the corner of the mouth.

ST5 Da ying: Anterior to the angle of the mandible on the anterior border of the masseter muscle in a groove-like depression when the cheek is bulged.

ST6 Jia che: One finger width anterior and superior to the lower angle of the mandible, at the prominence of the masseter muscle.

ST7 Xia guan: Anterior to the ear, with mouth closed, in the depression at the lower border of the zygomatic arch, anterior to the condyloid process of the mandible.

ST8 Tou wei: 0.5 cun within the hairline at the corner of the forehead, 4.5 cun lateral to the midline at DU24.

ST9 Ren ying: Level with the tip of the Adam's apple on the anterior border of the SCM. Avoid puncturing the common carotid artery.

ST10 Shui tu: Midway between ST9 and ST11 at the anterior border of the SCM.

ST11 Qi she: At the superior border of the medial end of the clavicle between the sternal head and the clavicular head of the SCM.

ST12 Que pen: At the midpoint of the supraclavicular fossa 4 cun lateral to the midline.

ST13 Qi hu: In the infraclavicular fossa, 4 cun lateral to the midline, below ST12.

ST14 Ku fang: 4 cun lateral to the midline in the first intercostal space.

ST15 Wu yi: 4 cun lateral to the midline in the second intercostal space.

ST16 Ying chuang: 4 cun lateral to the midline in the third intercostal space.

ST17 Ru zhong: 4 cun lateral to the midline in the fourth intercostal space at the center of the nipple. Contraindicated to needling and moxibustion.

ST18 Ru gen: 4 cun lateral to the midline in the fifth intercostal space.

ST19 Bu rong: 2 cun lateral to the midline lateral to RN14, 6 cun above the umbilicus.

ST20 Cheng man: 2 cun lateral to the midline lateral to RN13, 5 cun above the umbilicus.

ST21 Liang men: 2 cun lateral to the midline lateral to RN12, 4 cun above the umbilicus.

ST22 Guan men: 2 cun lateral to the midline lateral to RN11, 3 cun above the umbilicus.

ST23 Tai yi: 2 cun lateral to the midline lateral to RN10, 2 cun above the umbilicus.

ST24 Hua rou men: 2 cun lateral to the midline lateral to RN9, 1 cun above the umbilicus.

ST25 Tian shu: 2 cun lateral to the midline lateral to RN8 at the level of the umbilicus.

ST26 Wai ling: 2 cun lateral to the midline lateral to RN7, 1 cun below the umbilicus.

ST27 Da ju: 2 cun lateral to the midline lateral to RN5, 2 cun below the umbilicus.

ST28 Shui dao: 2 cun lateral to the midline lateral to RN4, 3 cun below the umbilicus.

ST29 Gui lai: 2 cun lateral to the midline lateral to RN3, 4 cun below the umbilicus.

ST30 Qi chong: 2 cun lateral to the midline lateral to RN2, level with the symphysis pubis.

ST31 Bi guan: With the thigh flexed, in the depression lateral to the sartorius muscle, directly inferior to the anterior superior iliac spine (ASIS).

ST32 Fu tu: 6 cun above the superior lateral border of the patella on the line connecting the ASIS.

ST33 Yin shi: 3 cun above the superior lateral border of the patella on the line connecting the ASIS found with the knee flexed.

ST34 Liang qiu: 2 cun above the superior lateral border of the patella on the line connecting the ASIS found with the knee flexed.

ST35 Du bi: Below the patella in a depression lateral to the patella ligament found with the knee flexed.

ST36 Zu san li: 3 cun below ST35, one finger width lateral from the anterior crest of the tibia, in the tibialis anterior muscle.

ST37 Shang ju xu: 3 cun below ST36, one finger width lateral from the anterior crest of the tibia.

ST38 Tiao kou: 5 cun below ST36, one finger width lateral from the anterior crest of the tibia.

ST39 Xia ju xu: 1 cun below ST38, one finger width lateral from the anterior crest of the tibia.

ST40 Feng long: 8 cun superior to the tip of the external malleous, one finger width lateral to ST38.

ST41 Jie xi: On the dorsum of the foot at the midpoint of the transverse crease of the ankle joint, approximately level with the tip of the external malleolus in a depression between the extensor digitorum longus and hallucis longus tendons.

ST42 Chong yang: On the dorsum of the foot, 1.5 cun inferior to ST41, in the depression between the second and third metatarsals and cuneiform bone. Avoid the dorsal artery when needling.

ST43 Xian gu: In a depression distal to the junction of the second and third metatarsal bones.

ST44 Nei ting: At the proximal end of the web between the second and third toes in the depression distal and lateral to the second metatarsodigital joint.

ST45 Li dui: 0.1 cun posterior to the corner of the nail on the lateral side of the second toe.

Spleen Meridian of Foot Tai Yin (SP)

Point locations:

SP1 Yin bai: 0.1 cun posterior to the corner of the nail, on the medial side of the great toe.
SP2 Da du: On the medial side of the great toe, distal and inferior to the first metatarsophalangeal joint in a depression at the juncture of the red and white skin.

SP3 Tai bai: Proximal and inferior to the head of the first metatarsal bone in a depression at the junction of the red and white skin.

SP4 Gong sun: In a depression distal and inferior to the first metatarsal bone at the junction of the red and white skin.

SP5 Shang qui: In a depression distal and inferior to the medial malleolus, midway between the tuberosity of the navicular bone and the tip of the medial malleolus.

SP6 San yin jiao: 3 cun directly above the tip of the medial malleolus on the posterior border of the tibia. Contraindicated to needling during pregnancy.

SP7 Lou gu: 6 cun from the tip of the medial malleolus on the line connecting the tip of the medial malleolus and SP9 on the posterior border of the tibia (3 cun above SP6).

SP8 Di ji: 3 cun below SP9 on the line connecting SP9 and the medial malleolus.

SP9 Yin ling quan: On the lower border of the medial condyle of the tibia, in the depression between the posterior border of the tibia and gastrocnemius muscle.

SP10 Xue hai: With the knee in flexion, 2 cun superior to the superior border of the patella, on the bulge of the medial portion of the quadriceps femoris muscle.

SP11 Ji men: 6 cun above SP10 on the line connecting SP12 and SP10.

SP12 Chong men: 3.5 cun lateral to the midline at RN2, in the inguinal region, on the lateral side of the femoral artery. Avoid femoral artery when needling.

SP13 Fu she: 0.7 cun laterosuperior to SP12 and 4 cun lateral to the anterior midline.

SP14 Fu jie: 1.3 cun below SP15 and 4 cun lateral to the anterior midline, on the lateral side of the rectus abdominis muscle.

SP15 Da heng: 4 cun lateral to the center of the umbilicus, lateral to the rectus abdominus muscle.

SP16 Fu ai: 3 cun above SP15 and 4 cun lateral to the anterior midline at RN11.

SP17 Shi dou: 6 cun lateral to the anterior midline in the fifth intercostal space.

SP18 Tian xi: 6 cun lateral to the anterior midline in the fourth intercostal space.

SP19 Xiong xiang: 6 cun lateral to the anterior midline in the third intercostal space.

SP20 Zhou rong: 6 cun lateral to the anterior midline in the second intercostal space.

SP21 Da bao: On the midaxillary line, 6 cun inferior to the anterior axillary crease. Midway between the axilla and the free end of the eleventh rib.

Heart Meridian of Hand Shao Yin (HT)

Point locations:

HT1 Ji quan: Center of axilla on the medial side of the axillary artery. Avoid axillary artery.

HT2 Qing ling: With the elbow flexed, the point is found 3 cun above the medial end of the transverse cubital crease in the groove medial to the biceps brachii.

HT3 Shao hai: With the elbow flexed, at the medial end of the transverse cubital crease.

HT4 Ling dao: With the palm facing up, the point is found 1.5 cun above the transverse crease of the wrist at HT7.

HT5 Tong li: 1 cun above HT7 on a line connecting HT3 and HT7.

HT6 Yin xi: 0.5 cun above HT7 on a line connecting HT3 and HT7.

HT7 Shen men: On the ulnar end of the transverse crease of the wrist, in the small depression between the pisiform and ulna bones.

HT8 Shao fu: With a fist made, where the little finger falls between the fourth and fifth metacarpal bones.

HT9 Shao chong: 0.1 cun posterior to the corner of the nail on the radial side of the little finger.

Small Intestine Meridian of Hand Tai Yang (SI)

Point locations:

SI1 Shao ze: 0.1 cun posterior to the corner of the nail on the ulnar side of the little finger.

SI2 Qian gu: With a loose fist made, the point is found on the ulnar side of the fifth digit, in the depression distal to the metacarpophalangeal joint, at the junction of the red and white skin.

SI3 Hou xi: With a loose fist made, in the depression proximal to the head of the fifth metacarpal bone, at the junction of the red and white skin.

SI4 Wan gu: On the ulnar edge of the palm, in the depression between the fifth metacarpal bone and the hamate and pisiform bones.

SI5 Yang gu: Near the ulnar end of the transverse wrist crease on the dorsal side of the hand in a depression between the styloid process of the ulna and the triquetral bone.

SI6 Yang lao: On the dorsal side of the wrist, in the bony cleft on the radial side of the styloid process of the ulna.

SI7 Zhi zheng: 5 cun above SI5 on a line connecting SI5 and SI8, between the anterior border of the ulna and flexor carpi ulnaris muscle.

SI8 Xiao hai: With the elbow flexed, in a depression between the olecranon process of the ulna and the medial epicondyle of the humerus.

SI9 Jian zhen: With the arm abducted, 1 cun above the posterior end of the axillary fold, posterior and inferior to the shoulder joint.

SI10 Nao shu: With the arm abducted, directly above SI9 in a depression inferior to the scapular spine.

SI11 Tian zong: In the depression of the infrascapular fossa, one-third the distance between the lower border of the scapular spine and the inferior angle of the scapula, approximately level with the T4 spinous process.

SI12 Bing feng: Above SI11 at the center of the suprascapular fossa, in a depression when the arm is lifted.

SI13 Qu yuan: On the medial extremity of the suprascapular fossa, about midway between SI10 and the spinous process of T2.

SI14 Jian wai shu: 3 cun lateral to the lower border of the spinous process of T1 (DU13).

SI15 Jian zhong zhu: 2 cun lateral from the posterior midline below the spinous process of C7 (DU14).

SI16 Tian chuang: On the lateral neck posterior to SCM, posterior and superior to LI18, level with the Adam's apple.

SI17 Tian rong: Posterior to the angle of the mandible in a depression on the anterior border of the SCM.

SI18 Quan liao: Directly below the outer canthus of the eye in a depression on the lower border of the zygoma. Contraindicated to moxibustion.

SI19 Ting gong: Anterior to the tragus and posterior to the condyloid process of the mandible in a depression formed when the mouth is opened.

Bladder Meridian of Foot Tai Yang (BL)

Point locations:

BL1 Jing ming: 0.1 cun superior to the inner canthus of the eye in a depression.

BL2 Zan zhu: In the supraorbital notch at the medial end of the eyebrow.

BL3 Mei chong: 0.5 cun within the anterior hairline directly above BL2 and 0.5 cun lateral to DU24.

BL4 Qu chai: 1.5 cun lateral to DU24 and 0.5 cun within the anterior hairline.

BL5 Wu chu: 0.5 cun above BL4 or 1 cun above the anterior hairline and 1.5 cun lateral to DU23.

BL6 Cheng guang: 1.5 cun posterior to BL5 and 2.5 cun above the anterior hairline, 1.5 cun lateral to the midline.

BL7 Tong tian: 1.5 cun posterior to BL6 and 4 cun above the anterior hairline, 1.5 lateral to the midline.

BL8 Luo que: 1.5 cun posterior to BL7, 1.5 cun lateral to the midline.

BL9 Yu zhen: 1.3 cun lateral to DU17, on the lateral side of the superior border of the external occipital protuberance.

BL10 Tian zhu: 1.3 cun lateral to DU15 and 0.5 cun above the posterior hairline, in a depression on the lateral aspect of the trapezius muscle.

BL11 Da zhu: 1.5 cun lateral to DU13, level with the spinous process of T1. (The distance from the midline to the medial border of the scapula is considered 3 cun.)

BL12 Feng men: 1.5 cun lateral to the midline, level with the spinous process of T2.

BL13 Fei shu: 1.5 cun lateral to DU12, level with the spinous process of T3.

BL14 Jue yin shu: 1.5 cun lateral to the midline, level with the spinous process of T4.

BL15 Xin shu: 1.5 cun lateral to DU11, level with the spinous process of T5.

BL16 Du shu: 1.5 cun lateral to DU10, level with the spinous process of T6.

BL17 Ge shu: 1.5 cun lateral to DU9, level with the spinous process of T7.

BL18 Gan shu: 1.5 cun lateral to DU8, level with the spinous process of T9.

BL19 Dan shu: 1.5 cun lateral to DU7, level with the spinous process of T10.

BL20 Pi shu: 1.5 cun lateral to DU6, level with the spinous process of T11.

BL21 Wei shu: 1.5 cun lateral to the midline, level with the spinous process of T12.

BL22 San jiao shu: 1.5 cun lateral to DU5, level with the spinous process of L1.

BL 23 Shen shu: 1.5 cun lateral to DU4, level with the spinous process of L2.

BL24 Qi hai shu: 1.5 cun lateral to the midline, level with the spinous process of L3.

BL25 Da chang shu: 1.5 cun lateral to DU3, level with the spinous process of L4.

BL26 Guan yuan shu: 1.5 cun lateral to the midline, level with the spinous process of L5.

BL27 Xiao chang shu: 1.5 cun lateral to the midline, level with the first posterior sacral foramen.

BL28 Pang guang shu: 1.5 cun lateral to the midline, level with the second posterior sacral foramen.

BL29 Zhong lu shu: 1.5 cun lateral to the midline, level with the third posterior sacral foramen.

BL30 Bai huan shu: 1.5 cun lateral to the midline, level with the fourth posterior sacral foramen.

BL31 Shang liao: In the first posterior sacral foramen.

BL32 Ci liao: In the second posterior sacral foramen.

BL33 Zhong liao: In the third posterior sacral foramen.

BL34 Xia liao: In the fourth posterior sacral foramen.

BL35 Hui yang: 0.5 cun lateral to either side of the tip of the coccyx.

BL36 Fu fen (AKA BL41): 3 cun lateral to the midline, level with the spinous process of T2 on the spinal border of the scapula.

BL37 Po hu (AKA BL42): 3 cun lateral to DU12, level with the spinous process of T3 on the spinal border of the scapula.

BL38 Gao huang shu (AKA BL43): 3 cun lateral to the midline, level with the spinous process of T4.

BL39 Shen tang (AKA BL44): 3 cun lateral to DU11, level with the spinous process of T5.

BL40 Yi xi (AKA BL45): 3 cun lateral to DU10, level with the spinous process of T6.

BL41 Ge guan (AKA BL46): 3 cun lateral to DU9, level with the spinous process of T7.

BL42 Hun men (AKA BL47): 3 cun lateral to DU8, level with the spinous process of T9.

BL43 Yang gang (AKA BL48): 3 cun lateral to DU7, level with the spinous process of T10.

BL44 Yi she (AKA BL49): 3 cun lateral to DU6, level with the spinous process of T11.

BL45 Wei cang (AKA BL50): 3 cun lateral to the midline, level with the spinous process of T12.

BL46 Huang men (AKA BL51): 3 cun lateral to DU5, level with the spinous process of L1.

BL47 Zhi shi (AKA BL52): 3 cun lateral to DU4, level with the spinous process of L2.

BL48 Bao huang (AKA BL53): 3 cun lateral to the midline, at the level of the second sacral foramen.

BL49 Zhi bian (AKA BL54): 3 cun lateral to the midline, at the level of the fourth sacral foramen.

BL50 Cheng fu (AKA BL36): On the posterior side of the thigh at the midpoint of the inferior gluteal crease.

BL51 Yin men (AKA BL37): On the posterior thigh, 6 cun inferior to BL50, on a line joining BL50 and BL54.

BL52 Fu xi (AKA BL38): With the knee in slight flexion, in the popliteal fossa, 1 cun superior to BL53 and on the medial side of the biceps femoris tendon.

BL53 Wei yang (AKA BL39): Lateral to BL54 at the popliteal crease and medially to the biceps femoris tendon.

BL54 Wei zhong (AKA BL40): Midpoint of the transverse crease of the popliteal fossa between the biceps femoris and semitendinosus tendons.

BL55 He yang: 2 cun directly below BL54, between the medial and lateral heads of the gastrocnemius muscle, on the line connecting BL54 and BL57.

BL56 Cheng jin: On the posterior leg, 5 cun inferior to BL54, at the center of the gastrocnemius muscle, along the line connecting BL54 and BL57.

BL57 Cheng shan: In a depression below the gastrocnemius muscle, 8 cun inferior to BL54.

BL58 Fei yang: 7 cun above BL60, on the posterior border of the fibula, about 1 cun lateral and inferior to BL57.

BL59 Fu yang: 3 cun directly above BL60.

BL60 Kun lun: In a depression between the tip of the lateral malleolus and the Achilles tendon. Contraindicated to needling during pregnancy.

BL61 Pu can: Posterior and inferior to the lateral malleolus, directly below BL60, in a depression on the lateral calcaneus.

BL62 Shen mai: In a depression directly below the lateral malleolus.

BL63 Jin men: Anterior and inferior to BL62, in the depression posterior to the fifth metatarsal bone.

BL64 Jing gu: Below the tuberosity of the fifth metatarsal bone at the junction of the red and white skin.

BL65 Shu gu: Posterior to the head of the fifth metatarsal bone at the junction of the red and white skin.

BL66 Zu tong gu: In a depression anterior to the fifth metatarsophalangeal joint.

BL67 Zhi yin: 0.1 cun posterior to the corner of the nail on the lateral side of the small toe. Contraindicated to needling during pregnancy.

Kidney Meridian of Foot Shao Yin (KI)

Point locations:

KI1 Yong quan: On the sole of the foot, in a depression when the foot is in plantar flexion at the junction of the anterior one-third and posterior two-thirds of line connecting base of second and third toes and the heel.

KI2 Ran gu: Anterior and inferior to the medial malleolus in a depression on the lower border of the tuberosity of the navicular bone.

KI3 Tai xi: In depression midway between the tip of the medial malleolus and the attachment of the Achilles tendon, level with the tip of the medial malleolus.

KI4 Da zhong: Posterior and inferior to the medial malleolus in a depression anterior to the medial attachment of the Achilles tendon.

KI5 Shui quan: 1 cun directly below KI3 in a depression anterior and superior to the medial tuberosity of the calcaneus.

KI6 Zhao hai: In a depression 1 cun below the tip of the medial malleolus.

KI7 Fu liu: 2 cun above KI3 on the anterior border of the Achilles tendon.

KI8 Jiao xin: 0.5 cun anterior to KI7, 2 cun above KI3, posterior to the medial border of the tibia.

KI9 Zhu bin: 5 cun above KI3 on the line drawn from KI3 to KI10 at the lower border of the gastrocnemius muscle.

KI10 Yin gu: At the medial side of the popliteal fossa when the knee is flexed, between the tendons of the semitendinosus and semimembranosus muscles level with BL54.

KI11 Heng gu: At the superior border of the symphysis pubis, 5 cun below RN8, 0.5 cun lateral to RN2. (RN8 is at the center of the umbilicus.)

KI12 Da he: 4 cun below RN8, 0.5 cun lateral to RN3.

KI13 Qi xue: 3 cun below RN8, 0.5 cun lateral to RN4.

KI14 Si man: 2 cun below RN8, 0.5 cun lateral to RN5.

KI15 Zhong zhu: 1 cun below RN8, 0.5 cun lateral to RN7.

KI16 Huan shu: 0.5 cun lateral to RN8 at the umbilicus.

KI17 Shang qu: 2 cun above RN8, 0.5 cun lateral to RN10.

KI18 Shi guan: 3 cun above RN8, 0.5 cun lateral to RN11.

KI19 Yin du: 4 cun above RN8, 0.5 cun lateral to RN12.

KI20 Fu tong gu: 5 cun above RN8, 0.5 cun lateral to RN13.

KI21 You men: 6 cun above RN8, 0.5 cun lateral to RN14. Avoid liver when needling.

KI22 Bu lang: In fifth intercostal space, 2 cun lateral to RN16. Avoid heart when needling.

KI23 Shen feng: In fourth intercostal space, 2 cun lateral to RN17. Avoid heart when needling.

KI24 Ling xu: In third intercostal space, 2 cun lateral to RN18. Avoid heart when needling.

KI25 Shen cang: In second intercostal space, 2 cun lateral to RN19. Avoid heart when needling.

KI26 Yu zhong: In first intercostal space, 2 cun lateral to RN20.

KI27 Shu fu: In the depression on the lower border of the clavicle, 2 cun lateral to the midline.

Pericardium Meridian of Hand Jue Yin (PC)

Point locations:

PC1 Tian chi: 5 cun lateral to the anterior midline or 1 cun lateral to the nipple in the fourth intercostal space. Deep needling not advised.

PC2 Tian quan: 2 cun below the anterior axillary fold between the two heads of the biceps brachii.

PC3 Qu ze: On the transverse cubital crease, on the ulnar side of the biceps brachii tendon.

PC4 Xi men: 5 cun above the transverse crease of the wrist PC7, between the palmaris longus and flexor carpi radialis tendons, on the line connecting PC3 and PC7.

PC5 Jian shi: 3 cun above the transverse crease of the wrist PC7, between the palmaris longus and flexor carpi radialis tendons, on the line connecting PC3 and PC7.

PC6 Nei guan: 2 cun above the transverse crease of the wrist PC7, between the palmaris longus and flexor carpi radialis tendons, on the line connecting PC3 and PC7.

PC7 Da ling: In the middle of the transverse crease of the wrist between the palmaris longus and flexor carpi radialis tendons.

PC8 Lao gong: On the transverse crease of the palm just below where the tip of the middle finger rests when a fist is made. Between the second and third metacarpal bones.

PC9 Zhong chong: At the center of the tip of the middle finger. For graphing measurement, 0.1 cun posterior lateral to the corner of the nail.

San Jiao Meridian of Hand Shao Yang (SJ)

Point locations:

SJ1 Guan chong: 0.1 cun posterior to the corner of the nail on the ulnar side of the fourth digit.

SJ2 Ye men: 0.5 cun proximal to the margin of the web between the fourth and fifth digits.

SJ3 Zhong zhu: With the fist clenched, on the dorsum of the hand between the fourth and fifth metacarpal bones in a depression proximal to the fourth metacarpophalangeal joint.

SJ4 Yang chi: On the transverse crease of the dorsum of the wrist between the tendons of the muscles extensor digitorum and extensor digiti minimi.

SJ5 Wai guan: On the dorsum of the forearm, 2 cun above SJ4 between the radius and the ulna.

SJ6 Zhi gou: On the dorsum of the forearm, 3 cun above the SJ4 between the radius and the ulna.

SJ7 Hui zong: One finger width lateral to SJ6 on the radial side of the ulna.

SJ8 San yang luo: On the dorsum of the forearm 4 cun above SJ4 between the radius and the ulna.

SJ9 Si du: On the dorsum of the forearm, 5 cun below the olecranon between the radius and the ulna.

SJ10 Tian jing: 1 cun superior to the olecranon in a depression formed with the elbow flexed.

SJ11 Qing leng yuan: With the elbow flexed, 1 cun above SJ10.

SJ12 Xiao luo: 5 cun superior to the olecranon on a line midway between SJ10 and SJ14.

SJ13 Nao hui: 3 cun below SJ14 on the posterior border of the deltoid muscle, on the line joining the olecranon and SJ14.

SJ14 Jian liao: In the depression posterior and inferior to the acromion process, about 1 cun posterior to LI15.

SJ15 Tian liao: Midway between GB21 and SI13 on the superior angle of the scapula.

SJ16 Tian you: Posterior and inferior to the mastoid process, on the posterior border of the SCM and level with BL10.

SJ17 Yi feng: Posterior to the lobule of the ear in a depression between the mandible and the mastoid process.

SJ18 Qi mai: At the center of the mastoid process at the junction of the middle and lower third of the curve formed by SJ17 and SJ20, posterior to the helix.

SJ19 Lu xi: Posterior to the ear at the junction of the upper and middle third of the curve formed by SJ17 and SJ20, posterior to the helix.

SJ20 Jiao sun: Directly above the ear apex, just above the hairline.

SJ21 Er men: With the mouth open, in the depression anterior to the supratragic notch and posterior to the mandibular condyloid process.

SJ22 Er he liao: Anterior and superior to SJ21, level with the root of the auricle on the posterior border of the hairline of the temple where the superficial temporal artery passes. Avoid artery when needling.

SJ23 Si zhu kong: In the depression at the lateral end of the eyebrow.

Gallbladder Meridian of Foot Shao Yang (GB)

Point locations:

GB1 Tong zi liao: 0.5 cun lateral to the outer canthus of the eye in a depression on the lateral side of the orbit.

GB2 Ting hui: Anterior to the intertragic notch at the posterior border of the condyloid process of the mandible with the mouth open.

GB3 Shang guan: Anterior to the ear, in the depression directly above ST7 on the upper border of the zygomatic arch.

GB4 Han yan: Within the hairline at the junction of the upper one-quarter and lower three-quarter distance between ST8 and GB7.

GB5 Xuan lu: Within the hairline midway between ST8 and GB7.

GB6 Xuan li: Within the hairline at the junction of the lower one-quarter and upper three-quarter distance between ST8 and GB7.

GB7 Qu bin: Within the hairline, anterior and superior to the auricle, about 1 cun anterior to TW20.

GB8 Shuai gu: Superior to the apex of the auricle, 1.5 cun within the hairline.

GB9 Tian chong: 0.5 cun posterior to GB8, 2 cun within the hairline directly above the posterior border of the auricle.

GB10 Fu bai: Posterior and superior to the mastoid process at the junction of the middle one-third and upper one-third of the curve between GB9 and GB12.

GB11 Tou qiao yin: Posterior and superior to the mastoid process at the junction of the middle one-third and lower one-third of the curve between GB9 and GB12 .

GB12 Wan gu: In the depression posterior and inferior to the mastoid process.

GB13 Ben shen: 0.5 cun within the hairline on the forehead, 3 cun lateral to DU4. Midway between ST8 and BL4.

GB14 Yang bai: On the forehead directly above the pupil, 1 cun above the midpoint of the eyebrow.

GB15 Tou lin qi: Directly above GB14, within the hairline, midway between DU24 and ST8.

GB16 Mu chuang: 1.5 cun posterior to GB15, 2 cun above the hairline and 2.25 cun lateral to DU22.

GB17 Zheng ying: 1.5 cun posterior to GB16, 3.5 cun above the hairline and 2.25 cun lateral to DU21.

GB18 Cheng ling: 1.5 cun posterior to GB17, 5 cun above the hairline and 2.25 cun lateral to DU20.

GB19 Nao kong: At the upper border of the external occipital protuberance, 2.5 cun lateral and level to DU17. Directly above GB20.

GB20 Feng chi: In the depression created between the origins of the sternocleidomastoid and trapezius muscles, at the junction of the occipital and nuchal regions. Lateral and level with DU16.

GB21 Jian jing: Midway between the spinous process of C7 (DU14) and the acromion process at the highest point of the trapezius muscle.

GB22 Yuan ye: With the arm raised, 3 cun below the axilla on the midline in the fourth intercostal space, below HT1.

GB23 Zhe jin: 1 cun anterior to GB22 in the fourth intercostal space, level with the nipple.

GB24 Ri yue: Directly below the nipple in the seventh intercostal space, inferior to LV14.

GB25 Jing men: On the lateral side of the abdomen, at the lower border of the free end of the twelfth rib.

GB26 Dai mai: Directly below LV13 at the free end of the eleventh rib level with the umbilicus (RN8).

GB27 Wu shu: On the lateral side of the abdomen, anterior to the ASIS, 3 cun below the level of the umbilicus, lateral to RN4.

GB28 Wei dao: Anterior and inferior to the ASIS, 0.5 cun anterior and inferior to GB27.

GB29 Ju liao: In a depression at the midpoint between the ASIS and the greater trochanter of the femur. Indications: cystitis, diarrhea, endometriosis, leg pain, leg paralysis, lumbar pain, orchitis, paralysis, sciatica.

GB30 Huan tiao: At the junction of the lateral one-third and medial two-thirds of the distance between the greater trochanter and the hiatus of the sacrum (DU2).

GB31 Feng shi: 7 cun above the transverse popliteal crease on the lateral midline of the thigh, where the tip of the middle finger touches when the patient is standing and the hands are at the sides.

GB32 Zhong du: On the lateral side of the thigh, 5 cun above the transverse popliteal crease between the vastus lateralis and biceps femoris muscles, 2 cun below GB31.

GB33 Xi yang guan: On the lateral side of the thigh, 3 cun above the transverse popliteal crease, in a depression superior and posterior to the lateral condyle of the femur, between the femur and the tendon of biceps femoris.

GB34 Yang ling quan: In a depression anterior and inferior to the head of the fibula.

GB35 Yang jiao: 7 cun above the tip of the lateral malleous on the posterior border of the fibula.

GB36 Wai qui: 7 cun above the tip of the lateral malleous on the anterior border of the fibula.

GB37 Guang ming: 5 cun above the tip of the lateral malleous on the anterior border of the fibula.

GB38 Yang fu: 4 cun above and slightly anterior to the tip of the lateral malleous on the anterior border of the fibula.

GB39 Xuan zhong: 3 cun above the tip of the lateral malleous in a depression between the posterior border of the fibula and the tendons of peroneus longus and brevis muscles.

GB40 Qiu xu: Anterior and inferior to the lateral malleous in a depression on the lateral side of the extensor digitorum longus tendon.

GB41 Zu lin qi: On the dorsum of the foot, in the depression between the fourth and fifth metatarsal bones.

GB42 Di wu hui: Posterior to the fourth metatarsophalangeal joint between the fourth and fifth metatarsal bones, on the medial side of the tendon of extensor digiti minimi.

GB43 Xia xi: On the dorsum of the foot between the fourth and fifth metatarsals, 0.5 cun proximal to the margin of the web at the junction of the red and white skin.

GB44 Zu qiao yin: 0.1 cun posterior to the corner of the nail on the lateral side of the fourth toe.

Liver Meridian of Foot Jue Yin (LV)

Point locations:

LV1 Da dun: On the lateral side of the great toe, 0.1 cun from the corner of the nail.

LV2 Xing jian: On the dorsum of the foot between the first and second toes, proximal to the margin of the web at the junction of the red and white skin.

LV3 Tai chong: On the dorsum of the foot in a depression distal to the junction of the first and second metatarsal bones.

LV4 Zhong feng: 1 cun anterior to the medial malleolus, midway between SP5 and ST41, in a depression on the medial side of the tendon of tibialis anterior.

LV5 Li gou: 5 cun above the tip of the medial malleolus on the medial side of the tibia.

LV6 Zhong du: 7 cun above the tip of the medial malleolus and posterior to the medial tibia.

LV7 Xi guan: 1 cun posterior to SP9, posterior and inferior to the medial condyle of the tibia in the upper portion of the medial head of the gastrocnemius muscle. In the depression of the medial border of the tibia.

LV8 Qu quan: When the knee is flexed, the point is found above the medial end of the transverse popliteal crease, posterior to the medial epicondyle of the tibia in a depression on the anterior border of the insertions of the semimembranosus and semitendinosus muscles.

LV9 Yin bao: 4 cun above the medial epicondyle of the femur, between the vastus medialis and sartorius muscles.

LV10 Zu wu li: 3 cun below ST30 at the proximal end of the thigh on the lateral border of the adductor longus muscle.

LV11 Yin lian: 2 cun below ST30, 2 cun from the midline at the proximal end of the thigh and on the lateral border of the adductor longus muscle.

LV12 Ji mai: 2.5 cun lateral and inferior to the superior border of the pubic symphysis. In the inguinal groove lateral and inferior to ST30.

LV13 Zhang men: On the lateral side of the abdomen below the free end of the eleventh rib.

LV14 Qi men: Directly below the nipple, 4 cun lateral to the midline in the sixth intercostal groove.

Ren Meridian (RN)

Point locations:

RN1 Hui yin: On the midline between the anus and the scrotum in males. Between the anus and the posterior labial commissure in females.

RN2 Qu gu: On the top of the notch at the center of the superior border of the pubic symphysis.

RN3 Zhong ji: 1 cun above RN2, on the midline, 4 cun inferior to the umbilicus.

RN4 Guan yuan: On the midline, 3 cun inferior to the umbilicus.

RN5 Shi men: On the midline, 2 cun inferior to the umbilicus.

RN6 Qi hai: On the midline, 1.5 cun inferior to the umbilicus.

RN7 Yin jiao: On the midline, 1 cun inferior to the umbilicus.

RN8 Shen que: At the center of the umbilicus.

RN9 Shui fen: On the midline, 1 cun superior to the umbilicus.

RN10 Xia wan: On the midline, 2 cun superior to the umbilicus.

RN11 Jian li: On the midline, 3 cun superior to the umbilicus.

RN12 Zhong wan: On the midline, 4 cun superior to the umbilicus.

RN13 Shang wan: On the midline, 5 cun superior to the umbilicus.

RN14 Ju que: On the midline, 6 cun superior to the umbilicus.

RN15 Jiu wei: On the midline, 7 cun superior to the umbilicus and inferior to the xiphoid process.

RN16 Zhong ting: On the midline, level with the fifth intercostal space at the sternocostal angle.

RN 17 Shan zhong: On the midline, level with the fourth intercostal space midway between the nipples.

RN18 Yu tang: On the midline, level with the third intercostal space.

RN19 Zi gong: On the midline, level with the second intercostal space.

RN20 Hua gai: On the midline, level with the first intercostal space.

RN21 Xuan ji: On the manubrium midline, 1 cun below RN22.

RN22 Tian tu: 0.5 cun superior to the suprasternal notch, at the center of the depression.

RN23 Lian quan: On the midline, in the depression superior to the hyoid bone.

RN24 Cheng jiang: In the depression at the center of the mentolabial groove, below the middle of the lower lip.

Du Meridian (DU)

Point locations:

DU1 Chang qiang: Midway between the tip of the coccyx bone and the anus with the patient lying prone.

DU2 Yao shu: In the sacral hiatus.

DU3 Yao yang guan: Below the spinous process of L4.

DU4 Ming men: Below the spinous process of L2.

DU5 Xuan shu: Below the spinous process of L1.

DU6 Ji zhong: Below the spinous process of T11.

DU7 Zhong shu: Below the spinous process of T10.

DU8 Jin suo: Below the spinous process of T9.

DU9 Zhi yang: Below the spinous process of T7.

DU10 Ling tai: Below the spinous process of T6.

DU11 Shen dao: Below the spinous process of T5.

DU12 Shen zhu: Below the spinous process of T3.

DU13 Tao dao: Below the spinous process of T1.

DU14 Da zhui: Below the spinous process of C7.

DU15 Ya men: 0.5 cun above the midpoint of the posterior hairline in a depression below the spinous process of C1.

DU16 Feng fu: 1 cun directly above the midpoint of the posterior hairline, directly below the external occipital protuberance. In the depression between the trapezius muscles of both sides.

DU17 Nao hu: Midway between DU16 and DU18, 1.5 cun above DU16.

DU18 Qiang jian: Midway between DU16 and DU20, 1.5 cun above DU17.

DU19 Hou ding: 5.5 cun above the midpoint of the posterior hairline. Midway between DU18 and DU20, 1.5 cun above DU18.

DU20 Bai hui: 7 cun above the midpoint of the posterior hairline, 5 cun above the midpoint of the anterior hairline, midway on a line connecting the apex of both ears.

DU21 Qian ding: 1.5 cun anterior to DU20. Midway between DU20 and DU22.

DU22 Xin hui: 2 cun posterior to the anterior hairline, 3 cun anterior to DU20.

DU23 Shang xing: 1 cun posterior to the anterior hairline, 0.5 cun posterior to DU24.

DU24 Shen ting: 0.5 cun above the midpoint of the anterior hairline.

DU25 Su liao: On the tip of the nose.

DU26 Ren zhong: At the junction of the upper and middle third of the philtrum.

DU27 Dui duan: At the junction of the upper lip and philtrum.

DU28 Yin jiao: At the junction of the gum and frenulum of the upper lip.

APPENDIX II
GLOSSARY

Ben (本)

Běn

Ben represents the dominant aspect of a disease process. It is a relative term in contrast with biao, including many meanings depending on the environment and references, such as causes, zheng, the primary, the interior, etc.

Treatment Based on CM Diagnosis (辨 证 论 治)

Biàn zhèng lùn zhì

Treatment based on CM diagnosis means establishing the treatment principles and methods based on a summary of all information relating to the patient's conditions, including signs, symptoms, etiology, pathogenesis, nature, location, stage, etc.

Biao (标)

Biāo

Biao represents the subordinate aspect of a disease process. It is a relative term in contrast with ben, including many meanings depending on the environment and references, such as manifestation, xie, the secondary, the exterior, etc.

Da Chang (大 肠)

Dà cháng

Da chang is one of the six fu organs. It relates to the large intestine, bowel movement, nose, nasal discharge, skin, transport, fluid metabolism, fei, hand yang ming channel, etc.

Dan (胆)

Dǎn

Dan is one of the six fu organs. It relates to the gallbladder, bile, eyes, tendon, tears, gan, foot shao yang dan channel, etc.

Du (毒)

Dú

Du has the following meanings: (1) pathogenic factors; (2) some zheng; (3) toxins from drugs or herbs.

Fei (肺)

Fèi

Fei is one of the five zang organs. It relates to the lung, nose, skin, qi, water metabolism, blood movement, da chang, hand tai yin channel, etc.

Feng (风)

Fēng

Feng has the following meanings: (1) one of the six yin; (2) some zheng.

Fu (腑)

Fǔ

Fu refers to the six hollow organs: dan, xiao chang, wei, da chang, pang guang, and tri-jiao. Their chief functions are to accept foods, absorb nutrients, and transport waste products.

Gan (肝)

Gān

Gan is one of the five zang organs. It relates to the liver, tendons, eyes, storage of blood, regulation of qi, dan, foot jue yin channel, etc.

Han (寒)

Hán

Han has the following meanings: (1) one of the six yin, belongs to yin xie; (2) some zheng.

Huo (火)

Huǒ

Huo has the following meanings: (1) some zheng; (2) some physiological factors; (3) some pathological factors; (4) one of the six yin, belongs to yang xie.

Jin (津)

Jīn

Jin has the following meanings: (1) components of body fluid; (2) saliva.

Lower Jiao (下 焦)

Xià   Jiāo

Lower jiao has the following meanings: (1) one of the tri-jiao referring to the lower portion of the body cavity; (2) some zheng.

Middle Jiao (中　焦)
Zhōng　jiāo
Middle jiao has the following meanings: (1) one of the tri-jiao referring to the middle portion of the body cavity; (2) some zheng.

Pang Guang (膀　胱)
Páng　guāng
Pang guang is one of the six fu organs. It relates to the bladder, urination, ear, bone, saliva, shen, and foot tai yang channel, etc.

Pi (脾)
Pí
Pi is one of the five zang organs. It relates to the spleen, limbs, muscles, digestion, blood retention, water metabolism, wei, and foot tai yin channels, etc.

Qi (气)
Qì
Qi has the following meanings: (1) the vital energy within the body; (2) the organ's functional activities; (3) the air inhaled and exhaled from the lung; (4) the body's defense system (zheng qi) and pathogens (xie qi); (5) some zheng.

Qi Heng Zhi Fu (奇　恒　之　腑)
Qí　héng　zhī　fŭ
Qi heng zhi fu refers to the fu organs, which are different from the six fu organs, including the nao, sui, gu, mai, dan, nu zi bao, etc.

Shen (神)
Shén
Shen has the following meanings: (1) the overall life processes of the human body; (2) the mentality, consciousness, and thinking processes.

Shen (肾)
Shèn
Shen is one of the five zang organs. It relates to the kidney, growth and development, control of urine and stool evacuation, respiration, water metabolism, pang guang, and foot shao yin channel, etc.

Shi (湿)
Shī

Shi has the following meanings: (1) one of the six yin belonging to yin xie; (2) some zheng.

Shi (实)
Shí

Shi has the following meanings: (1) some zheng; (2) some factors; (3) xie qi.

Shu (暑)
Shǔ

Shu is one of the six yin belonging to yang xie.

Six Yin (六 淫)
Liù yín

Six yin refers to the six pathogenic factors: feng, han, shu, shi, zao, and huo.

Sui (髓)
Suǐ

Sui is one of the qi heng zhi fu, including the bone marrow, spinal cord, etc.

Tai (苔)
Tāi

Tai refers to the layer covering the tongue surface.

Tan (痰)
Tán

Tan has the following meanings: (1) the mucoid substances secreted from the respiratory tract; (2) cause of a disease; (3) product of a disease; (4) some zheng.

Tri-jiao (三 焦)
Sān jiāo

Tri-jiao has the following meanings: (1) one of the six fu organs, including the upper jiao, middle jiao, and lower jiao; (2) the principle of treatment based on CM diagnosis in epidemic febrile diseases.

Upper Jiao (上焦)
Shàng jiāo
Upper jiao has the following meanings: (1) one of the tri-jiao, referring to the upper portion of the body; (2) some zheng.

Wei (胃)
Wèi
Wei is one of the six fu organs. It relates to the gastric cavity, mouth, flesh, saliva, digestion, pi, foot yang ming channel, etc.

Wei (卫)
Wèi
Wei has the following meanings: (1) a stage in the epidemic febrile diseases; (2) the body's defensive function; (3) wei qi circulating outside the vessels.

Xiao Chang (小　肠)
Xiǎo　cháng
Xiao chang is one of the six fu organs. It relates to the small intestine, tongue, vessels, sweating, xin, hand tai yang channel, etc.

Xie (邪)
Xié
Xie has the following meanings: (1) pathogenic factors; (2) pathological damages; (3) the six yin.

Xin (心)
Xīn
Xin is one of the five zang organs. It relates to the heart, vessels, blood circulation, control of mental activities, tongue, sweating, xiao chang, hand shao yin channel, etc.

Xin Bao (心 包)
Xīn bāo
Xin bao has the following meanings: (1) the outer layer of the xin functioning to protect the xin; (2) some zheng.

Xu (虚)
Xū
Xu has the following meanings: (1) some zheng; (2) pathogenic factors; (3) deficiency states.

Yang (阳)
Yáng
Yang is a Chinese philosophical term in contrast with yin. It relates to the active, moving, upward, etc., aspects of matters in the universe.

Yin (阴)
Yīn
Yin is a Chinese philosophical term in contrast with yang. It relates to the passive, still, downward, etc., aspects of matters in the universe.

Yin (饮)
Yǐn
Yin has the following meanings: (1) some zheng; (2) drinking; (3) drinks.

Ying (营)
Yíng
Ying has the following meanings: (1) essential substances in the channels and blood vessels; (2) movement; (3) one type of pulse; (4) some zheng.

Yuan Qi (元 气)
Yuán qì
Yuan qi is a type of qi inherited from the parents and reinforced after birth.

Zang (脏)
Zāng
Zang has the following meanings: (1) the five solid organs: gan, xin, pi, fei, and shen; (2) qi in the zang organs; (3) the outer physiological and pathological processes.

Zao (燥)
Zào
Zao has the following meanings: (1) one of the six yin belonging to yang xie; (2) some zheng.

Zheng (证)

Zhèng

Zheng is the summary of all information relating to the patient's conditions, including signs, symptoms, etiology, pathogenesis, nature, location, stage, etc.

Zheng (正)

Zhèng

Zheng has the following meanings: (1) general life function; (2) capability to resist diseases; (3) the normal four seasons.

Zhuo (浊)

Zhuó

Zhuo has the following meanings: (1) body discharges; (2) body wastes; (3) heavy fluids.

Appendix III
Index of Formulae

An gong niu huang wan (安 宫 牛 黄 丸)

Ān gōng niú huáng wán

Cow bezoar, curcuma root, rhinoceros horn, coptis root, scutellaria root, cape jasmine fruit, cinnabar, realgar, borneol, musk, pearl, gold foil.

An shen ding zhi wan (安 神 定 志 丸)

Ān shén dìng zhì wán

Poria, tuckahoe with hostwood, ginseng, polygalae radix, acoritatarinowii rhizoma, dragon's teeth.

Ba er dan (八 二 丹)

Bā èr dān

Gypsum ustum, hydrargyrum oxydatum crudum.

Ba zhen tang (八 珍 汤)

Bā zhēn tāng

Chinese angelica root, chuanxiong rhizome, white peony root, prepared rehmannia root, ginseng, bighead atractylodes rhizome, poria, prepared licorice root.

Bai he gu jin tang (百 合 固 金 汤)

Bài hé gù jīn tāng

Dried rehmannia, prepared rehmannia root, ophiopogon, fritillary bulb, lily bulb, Chinese angelica root, parched peony, licorice root, figwort root, platycodon root.

Bai hu tang (白 虎 汤)

Bái hǔ tāng

Wind-weed rhizome, gypsum, prepared licorice root, polished round-grained nonglutinous rice.

Bai tou weng tang (白 头 翁 汤)

Bái tóu wēng tāng

Pulsatilla root, phellodendron bark, coptis root, ash bark.

Ban xia bai zhu tian ma tang (半 夏 白 术 天 麻 汤)

Bàn xià bái zhū tiān má tāng

Pinellia tuber, gastrodia tuber, poria, tangerine peel, bighead atractylodes rhizome, licorice root.

Ban xia hou po tang (半 夏 厚 朴 汤)

Bàn xià hòu pǒ tāng

Pinellia tuber, magnolia bark, poria, perilla leaf.

Bao he wan (保 和 丸)

Bǎo hé wán

Hawthorn fruit, medicated leaven, pinellia tuber, poria, tangerine peel, forsythia fruit, radish seed.

Bao yin jian (保 阴 煎)

Bǎo yīn jiān

Dried Rehmannia, prepared rehmannia root, white peony root, Chinese yam, himalayan teasel root, baikal skullcap root, cork-tree bark, licorice root.

Bao yuan tang (保 孕 汤)

Bǎo yuàn tāng

Ginseng, astragalus root, Chinese cassia tree bark, licorice root, fresh ginger.

Bie jia jian wan (鳖 甲 煎 丸)

Biē jiǎ jiān wán

Turtle shell, belamcanda rhizome, scutellaria root, dried pillbug, fresh ginger, rhubarb, cinnamon twig, pyrrosia leaf, magnolia bark, Chinese pink herb, bignoniad, donkey hide gelatin, bupleurum root, dung beetle, peony, moutan bark, ground beetle, hornet's nest, niter, peach kernel, ginseng, pinellia tuber, lepidium.

Bu huan jin zheng qi san (不 换 金 正 气 散)

Bú huàn jīn zhèng qì sǎn

Magnolia bark, agastache, licorice root, pinellia tuber, atractylodes rhizome, tangerine peel, fresh ginger, Chinese date.

Bu yang huan wu tang (补 阳 还 五 汤)

Bǔ yáng huán wǔ tāng

Astragalus root, Chinese angelica root, red peony root, earthworm, chuanxiong rhizome, safflower, peach kernel.

Bu zhong yi qi tang (补 中 益 气 汤)
Bǔ zhōng yì qì tāng
Astragalus root, prepared licorice root, ginseng, Chinese angelica root, tangerine peel, cimicifuga rhizome, bupleurum root, bighead atractylodes rhizome.

Cang er san (苍 耳 散)
Cāng ěr sǎn
Magnolia flower, xanthium, dahurian angelica root, peppermint leaf.

Chai ge jie ji tang (柴 葛 解肌汤)
Chái gě jiě jī tāng
Bupleurum root, pueraria root, licorice root, scutellaria root, notopterygium root, dahurian angelica, peony root, platycodon root, fresh ginger, Chinese date.

Chai hu gui zhi gan jiang tang (柴 胡 桂枝 干姜 汤)
Chái hú guì zhī gān jiāng tāng
Bupleurum root, cinnamon twig, dried ginger, trichosanthes root, scutellaria root, ostreaeconcha shell, prepared licorice root.

Chai hu shu gan san (柴 胡 疏 肝 散)
Chái hú shǎū gān sǎn
Tangerine peel, bupleurum root, chuanxiong rhizome, nutgrass flatsedge rhizome, aurantii fructus, peony root, prepared licorice root.

Chu feng qing pi yin (除 风 清 脾 饮)
Chú fēng qīng pí yǐn
Orange peel, hypericum perforatum, saposhnikoviae radix, anemarrhena asphodeloides, weathered sodium sulfate, radix scutellariae baicalensis, radix scrophulariae, coptis, schizonepeta, rhubarb, balloonflower, rehmannia root.

Cong chi tang (葱 豉 汤)
Cōng chǐ tāng
Fistular onion stalk, pale fermented soybean, ginger.

Da bu yin wan (大补阴丸)
Dà bǔ yīn wán

Radix rehmanniae preparata, anemarrhenae, cortex phellodendri, the carapace, pig spinal cord.

Da bu yuan jian (大补元煎)
Dà bǔ yuán jiān

Ginseng, Chinese yam, rehmannia, eucommia, angelicae sinensis radix, corni fructus, wolfberry, cimicifuga, deer antler gelatin.

Da cheng qi tang (大承气汤)
Dà chéng qì tāng

Rhubarb, magnolia, citrus aurantium, Glauber's salt.

Da huang mu dan tang (大黄牡丹汤)
Dà huáng mǔ dān tāng

Rhubarb, cortex moutan, peach kernel, melon kernel, Glauber's salt.

Dan shen yin (丹参饮)
Dān shēn yǐn

Salvia, sandalwood, amomum.

Dan zhi xiao yao san (丹栀逍遥散)
Dān zhī xiāo yáo sǎn

Atractylodes macrocephala, bupleurum, Chinese angelica, poria cocos wolf, licorice, peony, gardeniae fructus, paeonia lactiflora.

Dang gui si ni tang (当归四逆汤)
Dāng guī sì nì tāng

Angelicae sinensis radix, cassia twig, peony, asarum, licorice, tetrapanax papyriferus, jujube.

Dao chi san (导赤散)
Dǎo chì sǎn

Rehmannia rehmanniae, akebia, radix glycyrrhizae uralensis shoots, bamboo leaf.

Dao tan tang (导 痰 汤)
Dǎo tán tāng
Pinellia, orange peel, poria, citrus aurantium, rhizoma arisaematis, licorice.

Di bi ling (滴 鼻 灵)
Dī bí líng
Centipeda, magnolia flower, ephedrine hydrochloride, glucose powder.

Di huang yin zi (地　黄　饮　子)
Dì huáng yǐn zǐ
Dried rehmannia glutinosa, morinda, cornus, dendrobium, cistanche deserticola, aconite, schisandra, cinnamon, poria cocos wolf, japonicus thunb, acorus calamus, polygala tenuifolia.

Di tan tang (涤 痰 汤)
Dí tán tāng
Poria, ginseng, licorice, orange peel, arisaema, pinellia, bamboo mushrooms, aurantii fructus, acorus calamus.

Ding chuan tang (定　喘　汤)
Dìng chuǎn tāng
Ginkgo, ephedra, coltsfoot flower, morus alba, perilla, licorice, almond, skullcap, pinellia.

Ding xian wan (定 痫 丸)
Dìng xián wán
Gastrodia, fritillaria, arisaema, pinellia.

E jiao ji zi huang tang (阿 胶 鸡 子 黄 汤)
Ē jiāo jī zǐ huáng tāng
Donkey hide gelatin, egg yolk, dried rehmannia root, white peony root, poria with hostwood, baked licorice, abalone, oyster, uncaria, caulis trachelospermi.

Er chen tang (二　陈　汤)
Èr chén tāng
Pinellia, dried orange peel, poris cocos wolf, licorice.

Er xian tang (二 仙 汤)

      Èr xiān tāng

Curculigo, epimedium, morinda, angelicae sinensis radix, cortex phellodendri, anemarrhena.

Er yan ling (耳 炎 灵)

      Èr yán líng

Rhubarb, scutellaria, coptis, phellodendron, sophora, borneol.

Er yin jian (二 阴 煎)

      Èr yīn jiān

Rehmannia, ophiopogonis radix, ziziphi spinosae semen, licorice, scrophulariaceae, berberine, poria, akebia.

Er zhi wan (二 至 丸)

      Èr zhì wán

Ligustrum lucidum, eclipta.

Fang feng tong sheng san (防 风 通 圣 散)

      Fáng fēng tōng shèng sǎn

Saposhnikoviae radix, fineleaf schizonepeta herb, hypericum perforatum, herba ephedrae, mint, rhizoma chuanxiong, radix angelicae sinensis, fried radix paeoniae alba, atractylodes macrocephala, gardenia, rhubarb, glauber's salt, gypsum, radix scutellariae, radix platycodi, licorice, talc.

Fu yuan huo xue tang (复 元 活 血 汤)

      Fù yuán huó xuè tāng

Bupleuri radix, trichosanthes root, angelicae sinensis radix, saffron, licorice, pangolin, rhubarb, peach kernel.

Gan lu xiao du dan (甘 露 消 毒 丹)

      Gān lù xiāo dú dān

Talc, scutellaria, artemisia capillaris, pogostemonis herba, weeping forsythia, acoritatarinowii rhizoma, white nutmeg, peppermint, akeriae caulis, rhizoma belamcandae, bulbus fritillariae cirrhosae.

Gan mai da zao tang (甘 麦 大 枣 汤)

      Gān mài dà zǎo tāng

Licorice, wheat, Chinese date.

Ge gen qin lian tang (葛 根 芩 连 汤)

Gě gēn qín lián tāng

Kudzu, licorice, scutellaria, coptis.

Ge xia zhu yu tang (膈 下 逐 瘀 汤)

Gé xià zhú yū tāng

Trogopterus, Chinese angelica, chuanxiong, peach kernel, moutan cortex, radix paeoniae rubra, radix linderae, corydalis rhizoma, licorice, cyperus, safflower, fructus aurantii.

Gua lou xie bai ban xia tang (瓜 蒌 薤 白 半 夏 汤)

Guā lóu xiè bái bàn xià tāng

Trichosanthes, allii macrostemonis bulbus, pinellia, Chinese liquor.

Guan zhong tang (贯 众 汤)

Guàn zhòng tāng

Japanese flowering ferm rhizome, melia, chenopodium ambrosioides, basil.

Gui pi tang (归 脾 汤)

Guī pí tāng

Atractylodes, Chinese angelica, poria, astragalus, longan meat, polygala, ziziphi spinosae semen, radix aucklandiae, baked licorice, ginseng, ginger, jujube.

Gui shao hong hua san (归 芍 红 花 散)

Guī sháo hóng huā sǎn

Chinese angelica, rhubarb, fructus gardeniae, skullcap, safflower, red peony, licorice, angelicae dahuricae radix, saposhnikoviae radix, dried rehmannia root, forsythia.

Gui zhi gan cao tang (桂 枝 甘 草 汤)

Guì zhī gān cǎo tāng

Cassia twig, licorice.

Gui zhi gan cao long gu mu li tang (桂 枝 甘 草 龙 骨 牡 蛎汤)

Guì zhī gān cǎo lóng gǔ mǔ lìtāng

Cassia twig, licorice, oyster, keel.

Gui zhi tang (桂　枝　汤)
Guì　zhī　tāng
Cassia twig, Chinese peony, ginger, Chinese date, licorice.

He ren yin (何　人　饮)
Hé　rén　yǐn
Tuber fleeceflower root, Chinese angelica, ginseng, dried orange peel, ginger.

He zi yin (诃　子　饮)
Hē　zǐ　yǐn
Terminalia chebula, almond, tetrapanax papyriferus.

Hei xi dan (黑　锡　丹)
Hēi　xī　dān
Black tin, sulfur, monkshood, psoaleae fructus, nutmeg, fennel, toosendan fructus, aucklandiae, lignum aquilariae resinatum.

Hong ling dan (红　灵　丹)
Hóng　líng　dān
Realgar, frankincense, moonstone, chlorite schist, myrrh, borneol, natrii sulfas, cinnabar, musk.

Hong you gao (红　油　膏)
Hóng　yóu　gāo
Petroleum jelly, gypsum calcined, hydrargyrum oxydatum crudum, east dan.

Hu qian wan (虎　潜　丸)
Hǔ　qián　wán
Cortex phellodendri, turtle shell, anemarrhena asphodeloides, radix rehmanniae, orange peel, paeonia lactiflora, cynomorium, tiger bone, ginger.

Hua gan jian (化　肝　煎)
Huà　gān　jiān
Ilex macropoda, dried orange peel, Chinese peony, male peony tree bark, gardenia, oriental water plantain, bolbostemmatis rhizoma.

Hua ji wan (化　积　丸)

Huà　jī　wán

Sparganium stoloniferum, curcuma, ferulae resina, pumice stone, concha arcae, cyperus rotundus, realgar, feces trogopterori, concha arcae.

Hua tan tong luo tang (化　痰　通　络　汤)

Huà　tán　tōng　luò　tāng

Pinellia, orange peel, citrus aurantium, chuanxiong, safflower, polygala, acorus gramineus, poria with hostwood, codonopsis, salvia, radix glycyrrhizae preparata.

Huang lian e jiao tang (黄　连　阿　胶　汤)

Huáng　lián　ā　jiāo　tāng

Berberine, scutellaria baicalensis, peony, donkey hide gelatin, egg yolk.

Huang lian di er ye (黄　连　滴　耳　液)

Huáng　lián　dī　ěr　yè

Berberine, borneol, glycerol.

Huang lian gao (黄　连　膏)

Huáng　lián　gāo

Berberine, scutellaria baicalensis, rhubarb, bee wax, sesame oil.

Huang lian jie du tang (黄　连　解　毒　汤)

Huáng　lián　jiě　dú　tāng

Coptis, scutellaria, phellodendron, gardenia.

Huang lian wen dan tang (黄　连　温　胆　汤)

Huáng　lián　wēn　dǎn　tāng

Berberine, caulis bambusae in taeniam, citrus aurantium, pinellia, orange peel, licorice, ginger, poria.

Huang qi jian zhong tang (黄　芪　建　中　汤)

Huáng　qí　jiàn　zhōng　tāng

Malt sugar, cassia twig, Chinese peony, ginger, Chinese date, astragalus root, licorice.

Huang qin tang (黄 芩 汤)

Huáng qín tāng

Radix scutellariae, radix glycyrrhizae uralensis, ophiopogon, morus alba, gardenia, hypericum perforatum, radix paeoniae rubra, radix platycodi, mint, fineleaf schizonepeta.

Hui yan zhu yu tang (会 厌 逐 瘀 汤)

Huì yàn zhú yū tāng

Peach kernel, safflower, licorice, balloonflower, rehmannia, Chinese angelica, figwort root, bupleurum, poncirus trifoliata, radix paeoniae rubra.

Huo xiang zheng qi san (藿 香 正 气 散)

Huò xiāng zhèng qì sǎn

Shell of areca nut, angelicae dehurieae radix, perilla, poris cocos wolf, pinellia, rhizoma atractylodis macrocephalae, dried orange peel, magnoliae officinalis cortex, platycodon grandiflorus, lophantus rugosus, licorice.

Huo xue li yan tang (活 血 利 咽 汤)

Huó xuè lì yān tāng

Chinese angelica, peach kernel, safflower, turmeric, rehmanniae radix, red peony, sophora tonkinensis, campanulaceae, silkworm, rhizoma belamcandee chinensis, licorice.

Ji sheng shen qi wan (济 生 肾 气 丸)

Jì shēng shèn qì wán

Radix rehmanniae preparata, dogwood, male peony tree bark, Chinese yam, poris cocos, oriental water plantain, Chinese cassia tree, monkshood, achyranthes bidentata, plantain seed.

Jia jian zhu jing wan (加 减 驻 景 丸)

Jiā jiǎn zhù jǐng wán

Wolfberry fruit, schisandra, plantain seed, mori fructus, sichuan pepper, rehmannia, Chinese angelica, dodder seed.

Jia wei er miao san (加 味 二 秒 散)

Jiā wèi èr miǎo sǎn

Phellodendri chinensis cortex, atractylodis rhizoma, Chinese angelica, achyranthes, menispermaceae, dioscorea collettii, turtle shell.

Jia wei jie geng tang (加 味 桔 梗 汤)

Jiā wèi jié gěng tāng

Platycodon grandiflorus, bletiliae rhizoma, citriexocarpium rubrum, lepidium apetalum seeds, licorice, fritillaria, coix, honeysuckle flower.

Jin gui shen qi wan (金 贵 肾 气 丸)

Jīn guì shèn qì wán

Radix rehmanniae exsiccata, Chinese yam, dogwood, poris cocos, male peony tree bark, oriental water plantain, cassia twig, monkshood.

Jin huang san (金 黄 散)

Jīn huáng sǎn

Rhubarb, phellodendri chinensis cortex, turmeric, angelica dahurica, rhizoma arisaematis, orange peel, eriocaulon herba, magnolia, licorice, trichosanthis.

Jin ling zi san (金 铃 子 散)

Jīn líng zǐ sǎn

Melia toosendan fruit, corydalis yanhusuo.

Jing fang bai du san (荆 防 败 毒 散)

Jīng fáng bài dú sǎn

Nepeta japonica, saposhnikoviae radix, angelica sylvestris, angelica sinensis radix, ligusticum wallichii rhizome, bupleurum chinense, peucedanum, platycodon grandiflorus, aurantii fructus, notopterygii rhizoma, menthae haplocalycis herba, poris cocos, licorice.

Jiu yi dan (九 一 丹)

Jiǔ yī dān

Gypsum, yellow elixir.

Ju yuan jian (举 元 煎)

Jǔ yuán jiān

Ginseng, astragalus, licorice root, cimicifuga, atractylodes.

Juan bi tong qiao tang (蠲 痹 通 窍 汤)

Juān bì tōng qiào tāng

Scutellaria baicalensis, coptis, coix, tetrapanax papyriferus, patchouli, loofah, acorus, magnolia, gleditsia, scorpio, radix glycyrrhizae uralensis.

Li zhong wan (理 中 丸)
     Lǐ   zhōng wán
Ginseng, ginger, atractylodes, licorice.

Lian li tang (连 理 汤)
    Lián   lǐ   tāng
Ginseng, ginger, atractylodes, licorice, poria, berberine.

Liang di tang (两 地 汤)
    Liǎng dì   tāng
Rehmannia root, ginseng, radix paeoniae alba, ophiopogon, cortex lycii radicis, donkey hide gelatin.

Liang fu wan (良 附 丸)
    Liáng fù   wán
Galangal, cyperus rotundus.

Liang ge san (凉 膈 散)
    Liáng gé   sǎn
Rhubarb, mirabilite, radix glycyrrhizae uralensis, gardenia, peppermint, radix scutellariae baicalensis, hypericum perforatum.

Liang xue xiao feng san (凉 血 消 风 散)
    Liáng xuè xiāo fēng sǎn
Rehmannia, Chinese angelica, fineleaf schizonepeta herb, cicada slough, sophora flavescens, tribulus terrestris, anemarrhena asphodeloides, gypsum, radix glycyrrhizae uralensis.

Ling gui zhu gan tang (苓 桂 术 甘 汤)
    Líng guì zhú gān tāng
Poria, cassia twig, atractylodes, licorice.

Ling yang gou teng tang (羚 羊 钩 藤 汤)
    Líng yáng gōu téng tāng
Antelope horn, uncaria, mulberry leaf, fritillaria, caulis bambusae in taeniam, dried rehmannia root, chrysanthemum, peony, poria with hostwood, licorice.

Ling yang jiao tang (羚 羊 角 汤)
Líng yáng jiǎo tāng

Antelope horn, morus alba, akebia, inula, polygonati odorati rhizoma, cimicifuga, poria with hostwood.

Liu jun zi tang (六 君 子 汤)
Liù jun1 zǐ tāng

Ginseng, rhizoma atractylodis macrocephalae, poria cocos wolf, roasted licorice, orange peel, pinellia ternata.

Liu mo tang (六 磨 汤)
Liù mó tāng

Betel nut, lignum aquilariae resinatum, radix aucklandiae, lindera aggregata, rhubarb, citrus aurantium.

Liu wei di huang tang (六 味 地 黄 汤)
Liù wèi dì huáng tāng

Rehmannia, cornus, yam, moutan cortex, alisma, poria.

Liu wei tang (六 味 汤)
Liù wèi tāng

Aconite, asarum, licorice, ginseng, dried ginger, rhubarb.

Long dan xie gan tang (龙 胆 泻 肝 汤)
Lóng dǎn xiè gān tāng

Bupleurum, alisma, plantago, akebiae caulis, dried rehmannia root, Chinese angelica, gentiana.

Lu feng ling yang yin (绿 风 羚 羊 饮)
Lü fēng líng yáng yǐn

Scrophularia buergeriana, saposhnikoviae radix, poris cocos, anemarrhenae rhizoma, scutellaria baicalensis, asarum, platycodon grandiflorus, antelope horn, plantain seed, Chinese rhubarb.

Ma huang fu zi xi xin tang (麻 黄 附 子 细 辛 汤)
Má huáng fù zǐ xì xīn tāng

Ephedra, monkshood, asarum.

Ma huang lian qiao chi xiao dou tang (麻 黄 连 翘 赤 小
Má huáng lián qiào chì xiǎo
豆 汤)
dòu tāng
Ephedra, forsythia, almond, red bean, jujube, morus alba, ginger, licorice.

Ma huang tang (麻 黄 汤)
Má huáng tāng
Ephedra, cassia twig, licorice, almond.

Ma xing shi gan tang (麻 杏 石 甘 汤)
Má xìng shí gān tāng
Ephedra, almond, gypsum, licorice.

Mai men dong tang (麦 门 冬 汤)
Mài mén dōng tāng
Ophiopogon, pinellia, ginseng, licorice, rice, jujube.

Pi pa qing fei yin (枇 杷 清 肺 饮)
Pí pá qīng fèi yǐn
Ginseng, loquat leaf, licorice, coptis, morus alba, cortex phellodendri.

Ping chuan gu ben tang (平 喘 固 本 汤)
Píng chuǎn gù běn tāng
Codonopsis, schisandra, cordyceps sinensis, juglandis semen, magnetite, lignum aquilariae resinatum, umbilical cord, fructus perillae, coltsfoot flower, pinellia, tangerine peel.

Pu ji xiao du yin (普 济 消 毒 饮)
Pǔ jì xiāo dú yǐn
Scutellaria baicalensis, berberine, dried tangerine peel, licorice, scrophulariaceae, bupleurum, campanulaceae, forsythia, radix isatidis, lasiophaera seu calvatia, arctium, mint, silkworm, cimicifuga.

Qi ge san (启 膈 散)
Qǐ gé sǎn
Radix glehniae, salvia miltiorrhiza, poria cocos wolf, bulbus fritillariae cirrhosae, curcuma, amomi shell, lotus leaf stem, rice spermoderm.

Qi ju di huang tang (杞 菊 地 黄 汤)

Qǐ jú dì huáng tāng

Wolfberry, chrysanthemum, rehmannia, cornus, yam, alisma, moutan cortex, poria.

Qi wei dou qi wan (七 味 都 气 丸)

Qī wèi dōu qì wán

Schisandra, dogwood, poria cocos wolf, cortex moutan, rehmannia, Chinese yam, alisma.

Qian chui gao (千 锤 膏)

Qiān chuí gāo

Castor bean, pseudomonas, rosin.

Qian gen san (茜 根 散)

Qiàn gēn sǎn

Radix rubiae, scutellaria baicalensis, donkey hide gelatin, meretricis concha powder, oriental arborvitae leaf, dried rehmannia, licorice.

Qian jin wei jing tang (千 金 苇 茎 汤)

Qiān jīn wěi jīng tāng

Reed stem, coix seed, melon kernal, peach kernel.

Qing chui kou san (青 吹 口 散)

Qīng chuī kǒu sǎn

Calcined gypsum, hominis urinae sedimentum, indigo, mint, phellodendron, coptis, fried moonstone, borneol.

Qing dai san (青 黛 散)

Qīng dài sǎn

Indigo, gypsum, talc, cortex phellodendri.

Qing dan tang (清 胆 汤)

Qīng dǎn tāng

Bupleurum, skullcap, gardenia, turmeric, citrus aurantium, rhubarb, lonicerae japonicae hos, artemisia capillaris, lysimachia christinae, coptis, mirabilite.

Qing feng san (清 风 散)

Qīng fēng sǎn

Chuanxiong, notopterygium, bupleurum, mint, saffron, Chinese angelica tail, campanulaceae, citrus aurantium, orange peel, licorice.

Qing jie tou biao tang (清 解 透 表 汤)

Qīng jiě tòu biǎo tāng

Cocumen tamaricis, kudzu root, cicada slough, cimicifuga fetida simpley, mulberry leaf, chrysanthemum, weeping forsythia, white honeysuckle flower, burdock, radix amebiae.

Qing jing san (清 经 散)

Qīng jīng sǎn

Cortex moutan, cortex lycii, radix paeoniae alba, radix rehmanniae preparata, herba artemisiae annuae, poria cocos wolf, cortex phellodendri.

Qing pi yin (青 皮 饮)

Qīng pí yǐn

Radix dick febrifugge, bambusa textilis, prunus mume, betel nut, amomum tsao-ko, licorice.

Qing re li yan tang (清 热 利 咽 汤)

Qīng rè lì yān tāng

Gypsum, skullcap, fritillaria, rhizoma belamcandae chinensis, scrophulariaceae, canarii fructus, trichosanthes, achyranthes, red peony, mint, licorice.

Qing re xie pi san (清 热 泻 脾 散)

Qīng rè xiè pí sǎn

Gardenia, calcined gypsum, berberine, rehmanniae radix, skullcap, poria cocos wolf.

Qing shu tang (清 暑 汤)

Qīng shǔ tāng

Forsythia, pollen, red peony, honeysuckle flower, licorice, talc, plantaginis semen, alisma.

Qing wei jie du tang (清 胃 解 毒 汤)
Qīng wèi jiě dú tāng
Cimicifuga, berberine, peony tree bark, rehmanniae radix, skullcap, gypsum.

Qing wei san (清 胃 散)
Qīng wèi sǎn
Cimicifuga, dried rehmannia root, Chinese angelica, berberine, cortex moutan.

Qing yan li ge tang (清 咽 利 膈 汤)
Qīng yān lì gé tāng
Peucedanum, saposhnikoviae radix, nepeta, forsythia, fructus arctii, radix sophorae tonkinensis, scrophulariae radix, gardenia, campanulaceae, licorice.

Qing yan xia tan tang (清 咽 下 痰 汤)
Qīng yān xià tán tāng
Scrophulariaceae, campanulaceae, licorice, burdock, fritillaria, trichosanthes, rhizoma belamcandae chinensis, nepeta, fructus aristolochiae.

Qing ying tang (清 营 汤)
Qīng yíng tāng
Rhinoceros horn, rehmannia, scrophulariae radix, bamboo leaf, ophiopogonis radix, salvia miltiorrhiza, berberine, honeysuckle flower, forsythia.

Qing zao jiu fei tang (清 燥 救 肺 汤)
Qīng zào jiù fèi tāng
Mulberry leaf, calcined gypsum, licorice, ginseng, black sesame seed, donkey hide gelatin, ophiopogon japonicus, almond, loquat leaf.

Qing zhang tang (清 瘴 汤)
Qīng zhàng tāng
Artemisia annua, bupleuri radix, poria, anemarrhena, orange peel, pinellia, scutellaria baicalensis, berberine, citrus aurantium, radix dichroae febrifugae, caulis bambusae in taeniam, talc, licorice, cinnabar.

Qu chong fen (驱 虫 粉)

Qū   chóng   fěn

Rangoon creeper, Chinese rhubarb.

Qu feng san re yin (驱 风 散 热 饮)

Qū   fēng   sǎn   rè   yǐn

Hypericum perforatum, arctium, notopterygii rhizoma, mint, rhubarb, radix paeoniae rubra, saposhnikoviae radix, Chinese angelica, licorice, gardeniae semen, ligusticum chuanxiong hort.

Ren shen yang ying tang (人 参 养 营 汤)

Rén   shēn   yǎng   yíng   tāng

Ginseng, Chinese angelica, astragalus, atractylodes, poria, cinnamon, rehmannia, schisandra, polygalaceae, orange peel, white peony root, licorice.

San huang xi ji (三 黄 洗 剂)

Sān   huáng   xǐ   jì

Rhubarb, phellodendri chinensis cortex, scutellaria baicalensis, sophora flavescens.

San zi yang qin tang (三 子 养 亲 汤)

Sān   zǐ   yǎng   qīn   tāng

Perilla, mustard seed, radish seed.

Sang bai pi tang (桑 白 皮 汤)

Sāng   bái   pí   tāng

Morus alba, fritillaria, almond, berberine, fructus perillae, pinellia, skullcap, gardenia.

Sang ju yin (桑 菊 饮)

Sāng   jú   yǐn

Almond, hypericum perforatum, mint, mulberry leaf, chrysanthemum, balloonflower, licorice, reed rhizome.

Sha shen mai dong tang (沙 参 麦 冬 汤)

Shā   shēn   mài   dōng   tāng

Glehnia littoralis, ophiopogon japonicus, trichosanthes root, lentil, rhizoma polygonati odorati, mulberry leaf, licorice.

Sha shen qing fei tang (沙 参 清 肺 汤)

Shā shēn qīng fèi tāng

Radix glehniae, astragalus, pseudostellaria heterophylla, albizia julibrissin, bletilla striata, licorice, balloonflower, coix, winter melon seed.

Shao fu zhu yu tang (少 腹 逐 瘀 汤)

Shǎo fù zhú yū tāng

Cumin, ginger, corydalis, myrrh, Chinese angelica root, cinnamon, red peony, pollen typhae, feces trogopterori.

Shao yao gan cao tang (芍 药 甘 草 汤)

Sháo yào gān cǎo tāng

Peony, licorice.

Shao yao tang (芍 药 汤)

Sháo yào tāng

Peony, Chinese angelica, berberine, betel nut, radix aucklandiae, baked licorice, rhubarb, scutellaria, cinnamon.

She gan ma huang tang (射 干 麻 黄 汤)

Shè gàn má huáng tāng

Belamcanda chinensis, Chinese ephedra, ginger, asarum, radix asteris, flos farfarae, jujube, pinellia, schisandra chinensis.

Shen fu long mu jiu ni tang (参 附 龙 牡 救 逆 汤)

Shēn fù lóng mǔ jiù nì tāng

Ginseng, aconite, keel, oyster, radix paeoniae alba, roasted licorice.

Shen fu tang (参 附 汤)

Shēn fù tāng

Ginseng, aconite.

Shen ge san (参 蛤 散)

Shēn gé sǎn

Gecko, ginseng.

Shen ling bai zhu san (参　苓　白　术　散)

Shēn　líng　bái　zhú　sǎn

Lotus, coix, amomum, campanulaceae, lentils, poria, ginseng, licorice, atractylodes, Chinese yam.

Sheng ji san (生　肌　散)

Shēng　jī　sǎn

Elephant hide, dragon's blood, pralloysitum rubrum, frankincense, keel, borneol, myrrh.

Sheng ji yu hong gao (生　肌　玉　红　膏)

Shēng　jī　yù　hóng　gāo

Licorice, dahurian angelica root, Chinese angelica, shikonin, ash, dragon's blood, calomelas.

Sheng mai san (生　脉　散)

Shēng　mài　sǎn

Ginseng, ophiopogonis radix, schisandra chinensis.

Sheng yu tang (圣　俞　汤)

Shèng　yú　tāng

Rehmannia, white peony root, rhizoma chuanxiong, ginseng, Chinese angelica, astragalus.

Shi pi yin (实　脾　饮)

Shí　pí　yǐn

Magnolia, atractylodes, papaya, aucklandiae, amomumtsao-ko fruit, areca seed, aconiti lateralis radix preparata, poria, ginger, licorice.

Shi xiao san (失　笑　散)

Shī　xiào　sǎn

Pollen typhae, feces trogopterori.

Shou tai wan (寿　胎　丸)

Shòu　tāi　wán

Dodder seed, taxillus chinensis, dipsacus, donkey hide gelatin.

Shu feng qing re tang (疏 风 清 热 汤)

Shū fēng qīng rè tāng

Fineleaf schizonepeta herb, saposhnikoviae radix, arctium, honeysuckle flower, forsythia, mori cortex, radix paeoniae rubra, radix platycodi, radix trichosanthis, radix scrophulariae, fritillaria, radix glycyrrhizae uralensis.

Shu zao yin zi (疏 凿 饮 子)

Shū záo yǐn zǐ

Rhizoma et radix notopterygii, betel nut, areca peel, poria peel, pepper, akebia, rhizoma alisma orientalis, phytolacca acinosa, red bean.

Shuang jie tang (双 解 汤)

Shuāng jiě tāng

Mint, fineleaf schizonepeta herb, mori cortex, honeysuckle flower, radix scutellariae baicalensis, gypsum, radix et rhizoma rhei, radix paeoniae rubra, cortex moutan.

Shui lun bing zhu fang (水 轮 病 主 方)

Shuǐ lún bìng zhǔ fāng

Codonopsis, fructus leonuri, wolfberry, dodder seed, Chinese angelica, safflower, rehmannia.

Shun qi dao tan tang (顺 气 导 痰 汤)

Shùn qì dǎo tán tāng

Orange peel, poria, pinellia, licorice, arisaema cum bile, radix aucklandiae, rhizoma cyperi, citrus aurantium.

Si jun zi tang (四 君 子 汤)

Sì jūn zǐ tāng

Ginseng, atractylodes, poria, licorice.

Si jun zi san (四 君 子 散)

Sì jūn zǐ sǎn

Codonopsis, atractylodes, poria, licorice.

Si ni san (四　逆　散)

_{Sì　nì　sǎn}

Licorice, citrus aurantium, bupleurum, peony.

Si shen wan (四　神　丸)

_{Sì　shén　wán}

Psoralea corylifolia, evodia fruit, nutmeg, schisandra chinensis.

Si wu xiao feng yin (四　物　消　风　饮)

_{Sì　wù　xiāo　fēng　yǐn}

Rehmannia, Chinese angelica, fineleaf schizonepeta herb, saposhnikoviae radix, radix paeoniae rubra, rhizoma chuanxiong, cortex dictamni, cicada slough, mint, angelicae sinensis radix, bupleurum.

Su he xiang wan (苏　合　香　丸)

_{Sū　hé　xiāng　wán}

Atractylodes macrocephala, radix aucklandiae, rhinoceros horn, cyperi, cinnabar, terminalia chebula, sandalwood, benzoin, aloe, musk, cloves, long pepper extract, borneol, styrax.

Su ye huang lian tang (苏　叶　黄　连　汤)

_{Sū　yè　huáng　lián　tāng}

Perilla leaf, Chinese goldthread rhizome.

Tai yi gao (太　乙　膏)

_{Tài　yǐ　gāo}

Scrophularia buergeriana, dahurian angelica, Chinese angelica, Chinese cassia tree, herbaceous peony, Chinese rhubarb, rehmanniae radix, momordica cochinchinensis, asafetida, calomel, tamaricis cacumen sophorae branch, roasted human hair, red lead, frankincense, myrrh, sesame oil.

Tai yuan yin (胎　元　饮)

_{Tāi　yuán　yǐn}

Radix ginseng, angelicae sinensis radix, eucommia, paeonia lactiflora, rehmannia, rhizoma atractylodis macrocephalae, roasted licorice, orange peel.

Tao hua tang (桃　花　汤)

Táo　huā　tāng

Red kaolin, dried ginger, rice.

Tao ren hong hua jian (桃　仁　红　花　煎)

Táo　rén　hóng　huā　jiān

Safflower, angelicae sinensis radix, peach kernel, cyperus, corydalis, radix paeoniae rubra, rhizoma chuanxiong, frankincense, salvia miltiorrhiza, citri reticulatae pericarpium viride, radix rehmanniae preparata.

Tian ma gou teng yin (天　麻　钩　藤　饮)

Tiān　má　gōu　téng　yǐn

Rhizoma gastrodiae, uncaria rhynchophylla, cassia, cape jasmine fruit, radix scutellariae baicalensis, achyranthes bidentata, eucommia, motherwort, taxilli herba, tuber fleeceflower stem, poria with hostwood.

Tian wang bu xin dan (天　王　补　心　丹)

Tiān　wáng　bǔ　xīn　dān

Ginseng, figwort root, radix salviae miltiorrhizae, poria, polygala tenuifolia, balloonflower, rehmannia, Chinese angelica, schisandra chinensis, asparagus cochinchinensis, japonicus thunb, arborvitae seed, semen ziziphi spinosae.

Tiao gan tang (调　肝　汤)

Tiào　gān　tāng

Chinese yam, donkey hide gelatin, Chinese angelica, herbaceous peony root, corni fructus, morindae officinalis radix, licorice.

Ting li da zao xie fei tang (葶　苈　大　枣　泻　肺　汤)

Tíng　lì　dà　zǎo　xiè　fèi　tāng

Lepidium apetalum seeds, jujube.

Tong qi san (通　气　散)

Tōng　qì　sǎn

Bupleurum, cyperus, ligusticum chuanxiong hort.

Tong qiao huo xue tang (通 窍 活 血 汤)
Tōng qiào huó xuè tāng

Herbaceous peony, ligusticum wallichii rhizome, peach kernel, red jujube, safflower, onion, ginger, musk.

Tong qiao tang (通 窍 汤)
Tōng qiào tāng

Saposhnikoviae radix, angelica sylvestris, ligusticum sinense, cimicifuga fetida simpley, kudzu root, ligusticum wallichii rhizome, atractylodis rhizoma, herba ephedrae, dahurian angelica, sichuan pepper, asarum, licorice.

Tong ru dan (通 乳 丹)
Tōng rǔ dān

Ginseng, astragalus, angelica sinensis, radix ophiopogonis, akebia, balloonflower, pig's feet.

Tong xie yao fang (痛 泻 药 方)
Tòng xiè yào fāng

Atractylodes macrocephala, Chinese peony, dried orange peel, saposhnikoviae radix.

Tong you tang (通 幽 汤)
Tōng yōu tāng

Chinese angelica, cimicifuga fetida simpley, peach kernel, safflower, licorice, dried rehmannia, ripe glutinous radix rehmanniae preparata.

Tou nong san (透 脓 散)
Tòu nóng sǎn

Astragalus, pangolin, ligusticum wallichii rhizome, Chinese angelica, Chinese honeylocust thorn.

Tou zhen liang jie tang (透 疹 凉 解 汤)
Tòu zhěn liáng jiě tāng

Mulberry leaf, chrysanthemum, mint, hypericum perforatum, arctium lappa, radix paeoniae rubra, cicada shell, viola yedoensis makino, coptis, saffron.

Tuo li xiao du san (托 里 消 毒 散)
Tuō   lǐ   xiāo dú   sǎn

Ginseng, astragalus, angelicae sinensis radix, peony, atractylodes, poria, honeysuckle flower, angelicae dahuricae radix, licorice.

Wei ling tang (胃 苓 汤)
Wèi   líng   tāng

Atractylodes lancea, orange peel, magnolia, licorice, rhizoma alisma orientalis, polyporus umbellatus, poria cocos wolf, rhizoma atractylodis macrocephalae, cinnamon.

Wen fei zhi liu dan (温 肺 止 流 丹)
Wēn   fèi   zhǐ   liú   dān

Terminalia chebula, licorice, platycodon grandiflorus, fish brain stone, nepeta japonica, asarum, ginseng.

Wen jing tang (温 经 汤)
Wēn   jīng   tāng

Evodia, Chinese angelica root, peony, ginseng, cassia twig, donkey hide gelatin, tree peony bark, ginger, licorice root, pinellia, ophiopogon.

Wen tu yu lin tang (温 土 毓 麟 汤)
Wēn   tǔ   yù   lín   tāng

Morinda, raspberry, atractylodes, ginseng, Chinese yam, medicated leaven.

Wu ling san (五 苓 散)
Wǔ   líng   sǎn

Polyporus umbellatus, rhizoma alisma orientalis, atractylodes macrocephala, poria, cinnamon twig.

Wu mei wan (乌 梅 丸)
Wū   méi   wán

Prunus mume, asarum, ginger, rhizoma coptidis, radix angelicae sinensis, radix aconiti lateralis, sichuan pepper, cinnamon twig, ginseng, cortex phellodendri.

Wu mo yin zi (五 磨 饮 子)
Wǔ   mó   yīn   zǐ

Radix aucklandiae, aloe, betel nut, citrus aurantium, lindera aggregata.

Wu pi yin (五 皮 饮)
Wǔ   pí   yǐn

Dried orange peel, poris cocos peel, ginger peel, mulberry root bark, shell of areca nut.

Wu wei xiao du yin (五 味 消 毒 饮)
Wǔ   wèi   xiāo   dú   yǐn

Honeysuckle flower, chrysanthemum indicum, dandelion, Chinese violet, radix semiaquilegiae.

Wu yao tang (乌 药 汤)
Wū   yào   tāng

Lindera strychnifolia, cyperus rotundus, Chinese angelica, aucklandiae radix, roasted licorice.

Xi jiao di huang tang (犀 角 地 黄 汤)
Xī   jiǎo   dì   huáng   tāng

Peony, rehmannia, peony tree bark, rhinoceros horn.

Xi jiao san (犀 角 散)
Xī   jiǎo   sǎn

Rhinoceros horn, coptis, cimicifuga, gardenia, herba artemisiae scopariae.

Xia chong wan (下 虫 丸)
Xià   chóng   wán

Meliae cortex, dryopteridis crassirhizomatis rhizoma, radix aucklandiae, peach kernel, ulmi macrocarpae fructus preparatus, betel nut, daucus carota, calomelas, dried rana limnocharia, quisqualis indica.

Xia ru yong quan san (下 乳 痈 泉 散)
Xià   rǔ   yōng   quán   sǎn

Chinese angelica, ligusticum wallichii rhizome, trichosanthes kirilowii root, herbaceous peony root, dried rehmannia, bupleurum chinense, ilex macropoda, rhaponticum uniflorum, platycodon grandiflorus, akebir quinata, dahurian angelica, hordei fructus germinatus, pangolin, cowherb, licorice.

Xian fang huo ming yin (仙　方　活　命　饮)

Xiān fāng huó mìng yǐn

Pangolin, licorice, saposhnikoviae radix, myrrh, herbaceous peony, dahurian angelica, Chinese angelica tail, frankincense, fritillaria, trichosanthes kirilowii root, Chinese honeylocust thorn, honeysuckle flower, dried orange peel.

Xiang sha liu jun zi tang (香　砂　六　君　子　汤)

Xiāng shā liù jun1 zǐ tāng

Ginseng, rhizoma atractylodis macrocephalae, poria cocos wolf, licorice, orange peel, pinellia, amomum villosum, radix aucklandiae.

Xiao ban xia tang (小　半　夏　汤)

Xiǎo bàn xià tāng

Pinellia ternata, ginger.

Xiao chai hu tang (小　柴　胡　汤)

Xiǎo chái hú tāng

Bupleurum, scutellaria baicalensis radix, ginseng, roasted licorice, ginger, jujube, pinellia ternata.

Xiao feng san (消　风　散)

Xiāo fēng sǎn

Chinese angelica, rehmannia glutinosa, saposhnikoviae radix, cicada slough, anemarrhena asphodeloides, sophorae flavescentis radix, flax, fineleaf schizonepeta herb, atractylodis rhizoma, fructus arctii, gypsum, licorice, akebia quinata.

Xiao jian zhong tang (小　建　中　汤)

Xiǎo jiàn zhōng tāng

Malt sugar, cassia twig, Chinese peony, ginger, Chinese date, roasted licorice.

Xiao ke fang (消　渴　方)

Xiāo kě fāng

Rhizoma coptidis, radix trichosanthis, lotus root juice, rehmannia root.

Xin jia xiang ru yin (新 加 香 薷 饮)

Xīn　jiā　xiāng　rú　yīn

Elsholtzia, honeysuckle flower, hyacinth bean flower, magnolia officinalis, hypericum perforatum.

Xing lou cheng qi tang (星 蒌 承 气 汤)

Xīng　lóu　chéng　qì　tāng

Arisaema cum bile, trichosanthes, rhubarb, mirabilite.

Xuan du fa biao tang (宣 毒 发 表 汤)

Xuān　dú　fā　biǎo　tāng

Cimicifugae rhizoma, kudzu root, peucedanum, platycodon grandiflorus, poncirus trifoliata, nepeta japonica, saposhnikoviae radix, peppermint, licorice, akebir quinata, weeping forsythia, burdock, almond, bamboo leaf.

Xue fu zhu yu tang (血 府 逐 瘀 汤)

Xuè　fǔ　zhú　yū　tāng

Chinese angelica, rehmannia, peach kernel, safflower, poncirus trifoliata, radix paeoniae rubra, radix bupleuri, licorice, balloonflower, chuanxiong, achyranthes bidentata.

Yang du nei xiao san (阳 毒 内 消 散)

Yáng　dú　nèi　xiāo　sǎn

Musk, borneol, hyacinth bletilla, turmeric, arisaematis rhizoma, manis squama, camphor tree ice, calomel, blue vitriol, verdigris, indigo naturalis.

Yang xin tang (养 心 汤)

Yǎng　xīn　tāng

Astragalus, poria, poria with hostwood, angelicae sinensis radix, pinellia, baked licorice, platycladi semen, polygala, schisandra, ginseng, cinnamon.

Yang yin qing fei tang (养 阴 清 肺 汤)

Yǎng　yīn　qīng　fèi　tāng

Rehmannia, ophiopogon root, licorice, mint, radix scrophulariae, fritillaria, peony tree bark, radix paeoniae alba.

Yi guan jian (一 贯 煎)

Yī guàn jiān

Radix glehniae, ophiopogon japonicus, rehmannia glutinosa, Chinese angelica, wolfberry fruit, melia toosendan fruit.

Yi wei tang (益 胃 汤)

Yì wèi tāng

Radix glehniae, ophiopogon, rock sugar, rehmannia, polygonatum odoratum.

Yin chen hao tang (茵 陈 蒿 汤)

Yīn chén hāo tāng

Artemisia capillaris, gardenia, rhubarb.

Yin chen wu ling san (茵 陈 五 苓 散)

Yīn chén wǔ líng sǎn

Artemisia capillaris, oriental water plantain, polyporus umbellates, poris cocos, atractylodes, cassia twig.

Yin chen zhu fu tang (茵 陈 术 附 汤)

Yīn chén zhú fù tāng

Artemisia capillaris, atractylodes, aconite, ginger, baked licorice, cinnamon.

Yin qiao san (银 翘 散)

Yín qiào sǎn

Hypericum perforatum, honeysuckle flower, balloonflower, mint, bamboo leaves, licorice, nepeta ear, semen sojae praeparatum, fructus arctii.

You gui wan (右 归 丸)

Yòu guī wán

Rehmannia, Chinese yam, dogwood, wolfberry, deer antler gelatin, dodder seed, eucommia, Chinese angelica, cinnamon, aconiti lateralis radix praeparata.

Yu lu san (玉 露 散)

Yù lù sǎn

Caleite, gypsum fibrosum, liquorice.

Yu nu jian (玉 女 煎)

Yù nü jiān

Gypsum, rehmannia, ophiopogonis radix, anemarrhena, achyranthes.

Yu ping feng san (玉　屏　风　散)

Yù　píng　fēng　sǎn

Saposhnikoviae radix, astragalus membranaceus, atractylodes macrocephala koidz.

Yue bi jia zhu tang (越　婢　加　术　汤)

Yuè　bì　jiā　zhú　tāng

Ephedra, gypsum, ginger, licorice, rhizoma atractylodis macrocephalae, jujube.

Yue hua wan (月　华　丸)

Yuè　huá　wán

Asparagus, rehmanniae radix praeparata, ophiopogon, rehmannia, Chinese yam, radix stemonae, adenophorae radix, fritillaria, donkey hide gelatin, poria, otter liver, panax notoginseng.

Yue ju wan (越　鞠　丸)

Yuè　jū　wán

Atractylodes lancea, rhizoma cyperi, medicated leaven, gardenia.

Zeng ye tang (增　液　汤)

Zēng　yè　tāng

Figwort, ophiopogon root, rehmannia root.

Zhen gan xi feng tang (镇　肝　熄　风　汤)

Zhèn　gān　xī　fēng　tāng

Achyranthes, ruddle, keel, oyster, testudinis carapax et plastrum, white peony root, scrophulariaceae, aspartame, meliae semen, malt, artemisia capillaris licorice.

Zhen ren yang zang tang (真　人　养　脏　汤)

Zhēn　rén　yǎng　zāng　tāng

Ginseng, Chinese angelica, atractylodes, nutmeg, cinnamon, licorice, peony, radix aucklandiae, myrobalan, poppy.

Zhen wu tang (真　武　汤)

Zhēn　wǔ　tāng

Poria, peony, ginger, atractylodes, monkshood.

Zheng qi tian xiang san (正 气 天 香 散)

Zhèng qì tiān xiāng sǎn

Lindera aggregata, dried tangerine peel, periliae folium, dried ginger.

Zheng rong tang (正 容 汤)

Zhèng róng tāng

Notopterygium, rhizoma typhonii gigantei, saposhnikoviae radix, gentiana, arisaema cumbile, silkworm, pinellia, licorice, ponderosa section.

Zhi bo di huang tang (知 柏 地 黄 汤)

Zhī bǎi dì huáng tāng

Radix rehmanniae preparata, cornus, Chinese yam, rhizoma alisma orientalis, poria cocos wolf, peony tree bark, rhizoma anemarrhenae, cortex phellodendri.

Zhi shi dao zhi wan (枳 实 导 滞 丸)

Zhǐ shí dǎo zhì wán

Rhubarb, citrus aurantium, medicated leaven, poria, scutellaria, coptis, atractylodes, alisma.

Zhu che wan (驻 车 丸)

Zhù chē wán

Ginger, Chinese angelica, rhizoma coptidis, donkey hide gelatin.

Zhu ye shi gao tang (竹 叶 石 膏 汤)

Zhú yè shí gāo tāng

Bamboo leaf, gypsum, pinellia, japonicus thunb, ginseng, licorice, rice.

Zuo gui wan (左 归 丸)

Zuǒ guī wán

Rehmannia, Chinese yam, wolfberry, dogwood, achyranthes, dodder seed, cervi cornus colla, testudinis carapacis plastri colia.

Zuo gui yin (左 归 饮)

Zuǒ guī yīn

Rehmannia, Chinese yam, wolfberry, baked licorice, poria, dogwood.

Supplement to Appendices

Appendix I. Acupuncture Points

Shi er jing: A general term including the 12 jing points of the 12 meridian channels.

Extra Points

Head and Neck

Sì shén cong: 4 points all at vertex of scalp, grouped around Du 20 and located 1 cun anterior, posterior and lateral to it.

Yìn táng: Midway between the medial ends of the two eyebrows.

Yú yāo: In the hollow, at the midpoint of the eyebrow, directly above the pupil.

Tài yáng: In the depression about 1 cun posterior to the midpoint between the lateral end of the eyebrow and the outer canthus.

ěr jiān: At the apex of the auricle.

Qiú hòu: At the junction of the lateral 1/3 and medial 2/3 of the infraorbital margin.

Bí tōng: at the highest point of the nasolabial groove ** No Moxa **

Jīn jīn (L)/ yù yè (R): on the veins of either side of the frenulum of the tongue — Jinjin is on the (L)eft side and Yuye is on the (R)ight side.

Bí tōng: 2 cun above GV 14 (C7) and 1 cun lateral.

ān mián: midpoint between TH 17 & GB 20 ** No Moxa **

Qiān zhèng: 0.5–1.0 cun anterior to the auricular lobe Indication: Deviation of the eyes and mouth, ulceration on tongue and mouth. Oblique 0.5–1.0.

Chest and Abdomen

Qipang: using the width of the mouth as the measure, construct an equilateral triangle with the navel at the apex, the two lower angles are Qipang ** No Needle in Pregnancy **

Zigongxue: 4 cun below the umbilicus, 3 cun lateral to the anterior midline ** No Needle in Pregnancy **

Back

Huatuojiaji: a group of 34 points, .5 cun lateral to the lower border of the spinous processes of T1-L5.

Dingchuan: .5 cun lateral to **GV 14** (C7).

Yaoyan: 3.5 cun lateral to the lower border of L4 (**GV 5**).

Shiqizhui (Josen): below the spinous process of L5 on the posterior midline.

Upper Extremities

Jianqian: midway between **LI 15** and the anterior axillary crease.

Erbai: 4 cun above the wrist crease, proximal to **PC 7** on both sides of the flexor carpi radialis.

Shixuan: tips of all 10 fingers ** No Moxa **

Sifeng: midpoint of the crease of each proximal interphalangeal joint ** No Moxa **

Baxie: on the dorsum of the hand, at the webs between each finger, at the junction of the red and white skin.

Luozhen: on the dorsum of the hand between the 2nd and 3rd metacarpal bones, about .5 cun posterior to the metacarpalphalangeal joint.

Yaotongxue: on the dorsum of the hand, midway between the transverse wrist crease and the metacarpalphalangeal joint, between both the 2nd and 3rd and 4th and 5th metacarpals (2 points on each hand).

Lower Extremities

Heding: in a depression at the midpoint and superior to the patella.

Xiyan: lateral (**ST 35**) and medial knee depressions.

Dannang Xue: 1–2 cun below **GB 34**.

Lan wei xue: 2 cun below **ST 36**. ** No Moxa **

Naoqing: 2 cun proximal to **ST 41** on the **ST 36-ST 41** line.

Shimian: in the center of the heel on the bottom of the foot.

Bafeng: on the dorsum of the foot between the web and metatarsophalangeal joint (4 points on each foot).

Neimadian: Found on the inside of the lower leg, 7 cun above the internal malleolus and 0.5 cun from posterior edge of the tibia.

Auricular Acupuncture Points

Auricular acupuncture points are listed in the following figure.

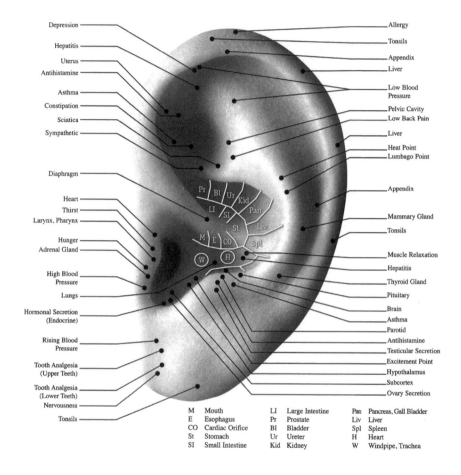

M	Mouth	LI	Large Intestine	Pan	Pancreas, Gall Bladder
E	Esophagus	Pr	Prostate	Liv	Liver
CO	Cardiac Orifice	Bl	Bladder	Spl	Spleen
St	Stomach	Ur	Ureter	H	Heart
SI	Small Intestine	Kid	Kidney	W	Windpipe, Trachea

Appendix II. Glossary

Bi (闭)

bì

It refers to several zheng in Chinese Medicine. (1) It refers to constipation and dysuria. (2) It refers to a zheng in stroke characterized by sudden falling into an unconsciousness state with lockjaw, clenched fists, constipation, dysuria, rigidity, and convulsion of limbs, etc. (3) It refers to a condition of lockjaw, clenched fists, constipation, dysuria, rigidity, and convulsion of limbs, etc in a feverish disease.

Chong (冲)

chōng

It refers to a name of meridian channels and collaterals. It is one of the eight extra channels and the sea of the twelve regular channels.

Huo (火)

huǒ

In addition to its other meanings in previous appendix, it also refers to fire.

Ji (积)

jī

It refers to abdominal mass at blood level.

Jia (瘕)

jiǎ

It refers to mass in abdomen at qi level.

Jing (精)

jīng

Jing has two meanings. (1) It refers to the essential substances constituting the human body including qi, blood, body fluid, essential substances from foods. Its main function is to maintain life activities. (2) It refers to essential substances for reproduction or congenital essence.

Ju (聚)

jù

It refers to abdominal mass at qi level.

Lao (劳)

Láo

Lao has to two meanings. (1) It refers to consumptive disease in Chinese medicine. (2) It refers to overexertion.

Ming men (命 门)

mìng mén

It has several meanings in Chinese Medicine. (1) It refers to the source of life processes and base of life. It's the root of primordial qi acting as the primary motivating force for the life activities. (2) It refers to the essence of close relation to human reproduction. (3) It refers to the acupoint of Du channel located at the spinous process between the 2nd and 3rd lumbar vertebra. (4) It refers to shimen acupoint on Ren channel. (5) It refers to Jingming point.

Nue (疟)

nuè

Nue refers to (1) a feverish disease with alternating chill and fever; (2) pathogen causing the feverish disease.

Qing (清)

Qing has several meanings in Chinese medicine. (1) It refers to the refined essence of food and water. (2) It refers to the cool air in fall. (3) It refers to the treatment clearing away the heat.

Ren (任)

rèn

It is a term in channels and collaterals referring to one of the eight extra channels.

San leng zhen (三 棱 针)

sān léng zhēn

It refers to a medical instrument in Chinese medicine made of stainless steel, with a cylindrical handle and a triangular sharp-edged body.

Tuo (脱)
tuō

It refers to several zheng in Chinese Medicine. (1) It refers to the zheng of severe exhaustion of yang qi and sudden departure of yin and yang characterized by cold limbs, excessive perspiration, unconsciousness, listlessness, pale complexion, vague and thread pulse, etc. (2) It refers to a zheng in stroke characterized by unconsciousness with the mouth open, eyes closed, hands relaxed, incontinence of urine and stools, snoring, etc.

Zhang (瘴)
Zhàng

Zhang refers to (1) moisture heat toxins, which can cause diseases; (2) one type of nue.

Zheng (癥)
Zhēng

It refers to mass in abdomen at blood level.

Zhi (志)
Zhì

Zhi refers to a mental activity in human body, characterized by being unswervingly faithful, and is related to kidney functions.

Appendix III. Index of Formulae

Ba zheng san (八 正 散)

bā zhèng sàn

Plantago, Dianthi herba, Polygonum aviculare, talc, mountain gardenia, Glycyrrhizae radix praeparata cum melle, Akebia, rhubarb, Junci medulia

Bai yu gao (白 玉 膏)

bái yù gāo

Lithargyrum, bees wax, frankincense, myrrh, elephant hide, insect wax, Calomelas

Bi xie fen qing yin (萆 薢 分 清 饮)

bì xiè fèn qīng yǐn

Longan kernel, dioscorea collettii, Acori tatarinowii rhizoma, Linderae radix

Bi xie hua du tang (萆 薢 化 毒 汤)

bì xiè huà dú tāng

Dioscorea collettii, Angelicae sinensis radix, Moutan cortex

Bi xie shen shi tang (萆 薢 渗 湿 汤)

bì xiè shèn shī tāng

Dioscorea collettii, Coix, smilax glabra Roxb, talc, tree Peony bark, alisma, Phellodendri chinensis cortex, Stachyuri

Bu fei tang (补 肺 汤)

bǔ fèi tāng

Ginseng, astragalus, schisandra, Rehmannia, Morus alba, Aster

Bu qi yun pi tang (补 气 运 脾 汤)

bǔ qì yùn pí tāng

Ginseng, rhizoma atractylodis macrocephalae, Orange peel, Poria, Astragalus, Amomum villosum, Radix glycyrrhiza uralensis

Chai hu jie nue yin (柴 胡 截 疟 饮)

chái hú jié nuè yǐn

Bupleurum, Scutellaria, Ginseng, Pinellia, licorice, ginger, Dichroae radix, betel nut, ebony, peach kernel.

Chai hu qing gan tang (柴 胡 清 肝 汤)
chái hú qīng gān tāng

Rhizome of Ligusticum wallichii, Angelicae sinensis radix, root of herbaceous peony, dried rehmannia, bupleurum chinensis, Scutellariae radix, mountain gardeniae, root of trichosanthes kirilowii, Saposhnikoviae radix, burdock, weeping forsythia, licorice

Chan su he ji (蟾 酥 合 剂)
chán sū hé jì

Bufonis venenum, realgar, basic cupric carbonate, Copperas, Calomelas, frankincense, myrrh, calcined alum, dried snail, musk, Dragon's blood, and tetranychus cinnabarinus, calamine, calcined calcitum, borax, rush pith ash

Chen xiang san (沉 香 散)
chén xiāng sàn

Aloes, Pyrrosiae folim, talc, vaccaria, Angelica, Malvae fructus, White Peony root, liquorice, orange peel

Cheng shi bi xie fen qing yin (程 氏 萆 薢 分 清 饮)
chéng shì bì xiè fèn qīng yǐn

Dioscorea collettii, Plantago, Poria, lotus, Acori tatarinowii, phellodendron, Salvia, Atractylodes

Cheng shi sheng tie luo yin (程 氏 生 铁 落 饮)
chéng shì shēng tiě luò yǐn

Ferrosic oxide, Uncaria, Arisaema cum bile, Fritillaria, Ctri exocarpium rubrum, Poria, Acorus gramineus, Radix polygalae, Poria with hostwood, tetranychus cinnabarinus, Asparagi radix, ophiopogon root, Forsythiae fructus, Scrophulariae radix, cinnabar

Chong he gao (冲 和 膏)
chōng hé gāo

Radix paeoniae Rubra, Radix angelicae dahuricae, Saposhnikoviae radix, Angelicae pbescentis radix, Borneol, Acorus gramineus

Chu shi wei ling tang (除 湿 胃 苓 汤)

chú shī wèi líng tāng

Atractylodes lancea, Magnoliae officinalis cortex, orange peel, Polyporus umbellatus, alisma, red Poria, rhizoma atractylodis macrocephalae, talc, Saposhnikoviae radix, mountainsgardenia, akebia, cinnamon, licorice

Chun ze tang (春 泽 汤)

chūn zé tāng

Alisma orientalis, Polyporus, Tuckahoe, rhizoma atractylodis macrocephalae, Cinnamomi cortex, ginseng, Radix bupleuri, Ophiopogonis radix

Cong gui ta zhong tang (葱 归 溻 肿 汤)

cōng guī tā zhǒng tāng

Angelica sinensis, Radix glycyrrhiza uralensis, Radix angelicae pubescentis, Dahurian angelica root, onion

Da chai hu tang (大 柴 胡 汤)

dà chái hú tāng

Radix bupleuri, Radix scutellariae, Paeonia lactiflora, pinellia tuber, ginger, citrus aurantium, jujube

Da fen qing yin (大 分 清 饮)

dà fèn qīng yǐn

Poria, alisma, akebia, Polyporus umbellatus, gardenia, Poncirus trifoliata, plantain

Da huang fu zi tang (大 黄 附 子 汤)

dà huáng fù zǐ tāng

Rhubarb, Aconiti lateralis radix praeparata, asarum

Dai ge san (黛 蛤 散)

dài gé sàn

Indigo naturalis, clam shell

Dai di dang wan (代 抵 当 丸)

dài dǐ dāng wán

Rhubarb, natrii sulfas, Peach kernel, Angelica sinensis radix, rehmannia, Manis squama, cinnamon

Dang gui yin zi (当 归 饮 子)

dāng guī yǐn zǐ

Angelicae sinensis radix, rehmannia root, Radix paeoniae Alba, Chuanxiong rhizoma, Radix polygoni multiflori, Schizonepetae herba, Saposhnikoviae radix, Thibuli fructus, Astragalus, licorice

Dian dao san (颠 倒 散)

diān dǎo sàn

Rhubarb, sulfur

Dian kuang meng xing tang (癫 狂 梦 醒 汤)

diān kuáng mèng xǐng tāng

Peach kernel, Radix bupleuri, Cyperi rhizoma, akebia Quinata, Radix paeoniae Rubra, rhizoma pinelliae, Arecae peel, Citri reticulatae pericarpium viride, Citri reticulatae pericarpium, Mori cortex, perilla, licorice

Ding kuang zhu yu tang (定 狂 逐 瘀 汤)

dìng kuáng zhú yū tāng

Salviae miltiorrhizae radix, amber powder, bupleurum root, Peach kernel, Carthami flos, Radix paeoniae Rubra, rhizoma acori tatarinowii, Rhei radix, Curcumae radix, Cyperi rhizoma

Er bai san (二 白 散)

èr bái sàn

Arisaematis rhizoma, Fritillaria

Er miao wan (二 妙 丸)

èr miào wán

Atractylodis rhizome, Phellodendri chinensis cortex

Fu fang tu jin pi ding (复 方 土 槿 皮 酊)

fù fāng tǔ jǐn pí dǐng

Pseudolaricis cortex, benzoic acid, salicylic acid

Fu zi li zhong tang (附 子 理 中 汤)

fù zǐ lǐ zhōng tāng

Aconite, codonopsis pilosula, atractylodes macrocephala koidz, dry ginger, licorice

Fu zi li zhong wan (附 子 理 中 丸)

fù   zǐ   lǐ   zhōng   wán

Aconite, codonopsis pilosula, atractylodes macrocephala koidz, dry ginger, licorice

Gao lin tang (膏 淋 汤)

gāo   lín   tāng

Chinese yam, Euryales semen, keel, oyster, Rehmanniae radix, codonopsis pilosula, root of herbaceous peony

Gua lou niu bang tang (瓜 蒌 牛 蒡 汤)

guā   lóu   niú   bàng   tāng

Chinese trichosanthes kernel, burdock, root of trichosanthes kirilowii, Scutellariae radix, mountain gardeniae, honey suckle, weeping forsythia, Chinese honey locust thorn, ilex macropoda, dried orange peel, bupleurum chinensis, licorice

Gua lou xie bai bai jiu tang (瓜 蒌 薤 白 白 酒 汤)

guā   lóu   xiè   bái   bái   jiǔ   tāng

Trichosanthes real, bulbus allii macrostemi, liquor

Gui she san (桂 麝 散)

guì   shè   sàn

Ephedra, asarum, cinnamon, Gleditsiae fructus, Pinellia ternate, cloves, Arisaematis rhizoma, musk, Borneol

Hai zao yu hu tang (海 藻 玉 壶 汤)

hǎi   zǎo   yù   hú   tāng

Sargassum, fritillaria, dried orange peel, Laminariae thallus, ilex macropoda, rhizome of Ligusticum wallichii, Angelicae sinensis radix, weeping forsythia, pinellia, licorice, angelica

Hei tui xiao (黑 退 消)

hēi   tuì   xiāo

Aconiti radix, Aconiti kusnezoffii radix, Arisaematis rhizoma, pinellia, magnet, male clove, Cinnamomi cortex, frankincense, myrrh, fried Nardostachys chinensis radix, sal ammoniac, borneol, musk

Hu po yang xin dan (琥 珀 养 心 丹)

hǔ pò yǎng xīn dān

Bovis calculus, coptis, ginseng, Radix rehmanniae, tetranychus cinnabarinus, amber fossil teeth, spine date seed, seed of Oriental arborvitae, Radix polygalae, Acorus, Poria with hostwood

Hua jian er chen wan (化 坚 二 陈 丸)

huà jiān èr chén wán

Citrus peel, Pinellia, Poria, Bombyx batryticatus, Coptidis rhizoma, licorice

Huai jiao di yu wan (槐 角 地 榆 丸)

huái jiǎo dì yú wán

Sophorae fructus, white peony root, fried Fructus, Nepeta, Burnet carbon Tsubaki leather, gardenia, skullcap, Rehmanniae

Huai jiao wan (槐 角 丸)

huái jiǎo wán

Sophorae fructus, the garden burnet, Scutellariae radix, Saposhnikoviae radix, Angelicae sinensis radix

Huan shao dan (还 少 丹)

huán shào dān

Chinese yam, Achyranthes bidentata, dogwood, white Tuckahoe, schisandra chinensis, Cistanche deserticola, Acorus, Radix morindae officinalis, Radix polygalae, eucommia ulmoides, fructus broussonetiae, fennel, fructus lycii, Radix rehmanniae Preparata

Huang qi tang (黄 芪 汤)

huáng qí tāng

Astragalus, seed of hemp, white bee honey, orange peel

Scutellariae radix qing fei yin (黄 芩 清 肺 饮)

huáng qín qīng fèi yǐn

Chuanxiong rhizoma, Angelica sinensis, Radix paeoniae Rubra, Saposhnikoviae radix, Rehmanniae radix, Puerariae lobatae radix, Radix trichosanthis, Forsythiae fructus, safflower, scutellaria, mint

Huang qin xie bai san (黄 芩 泻 白 散)

huáng   qín   xiè   bái   sàn

Scutellariae radix, Mori cortex, Cortex lycii, Radix glycyrrhiza uralensis

Hui yang yu long gao (回 阳 玉 龙 膏)

huí   yáng   yù   lóng   gāo

Aconitum, Arisaematis rhizoma, ginger, Angelica dahurica, Radix paeoniae Rubra, cinnamon

Hui zao san (灰 皂 散)

huī   zào   sàn

Kiln lime, natural water from crystal soda, red lead

Huo xue san yu tang (活 血 散 瘀 汤)

huó   xuè   sàn   yū   tāng

Rhizome of Ligusticum wallichii, Angelicae sinensis radix, herbaceous peony, sappan caesalpinia, Moutan cortex, Chinese trichosanthes kernel, peach kernel, betel nut, Chinese rhubarb

Ji chuan jian (济 川 煎)

jì   chuān   jiān

Angelica sinensis, Radix achyranthis bidentatae, Cistanche deserticola, rhizoma alisma orientalis, Cimicifuga, fructus aurantii

Jin huang gao (金 黄 膏)

jīn   huáng   gāo

Root of trichosanthes kirilowii, Curcumae longae rhizoma, Angelicae dahuricae radix, Atractylodis rhizoma, Arisaematis rhizoma, licorice, Chinese rhubarb, Phellodendri chinensis cortex, Magnoliae officinalis cortexe, dried orange peel, sesame oil, red lead

Jin suo gu jing wan (金 锁 固 精 丸)

jīn   suǒ   gù   jīng   wán

Tribuli fructus, euryale ferox, Lotus, keel, Oyster

Jin yin hua lu (金 银 花 露)

jīn   yín   huā   lù

Honeysuckle

Jiu hua gao (九 华 膏)

jiǔ   huá   gāo

Talc, borax, Fritillaria, Vermilion, keel, borneol

Ju he wan (橘 核 丸)

jú   hé   wán

Orange core, seaweed, Eckloniae thallus, laminaria japonica, Chinaberry fruit, Peach kernel, Magnoliae officinalis cortex officinalis, akebia Quinata, citrus aurantium, rhizoma corydalis, Cinnamomi cortex, costus root

Kai yu san (开 郁 散)

kāi   yù   sàn

White Peony root, Angelicae sinensis radix, white mustard, Radix bupleuri, Glycyrrhizae radix praeparata cum melle, Scorpion, rhizoma atractylodis macrocephalae, Poria, Curcuma, Cyperus, Semiaquilegiae herba

Ku shen tang (苦 参 汤)

kǔ   shēn   tāng

Radix sophorae flavescentis, Radix scutellariae, rehmannia

Ku zhi san (枯 痔 散)

kū   zhì   sàn

Natrii sulfas, potassium alum, bright realgar

Li zhong tang (理 中 汤)

lǐ   zhōng   tāng

Ginseng, ginger, licorice, Atractylodes

Liang xue di huang tang (凉 血 地 黄 汤)

liáng   xuè   dì   huáng   tāng

Scutellariae radix, Herba schizonepetae Spike, Viticisfructus, Phellodendri chinensis cortex, anemarrhena asphodeloides, ligusticum, asarum, Chuanxiong rhizoma rhizoma, rhizoma coptidis, rhizoma et radix notopterygii, Radix bupleuri, Cimicifuga, Saposhnikoviae radix, rehmannia, Angelicae sinensis radix, licorice, Carthami flos

Liu huang ruan gao (硫 磺 软 膏)

liú   huáng   ruǎn   gāo

Zinc oxide, sublimated sulfur

Liu wei di huang wan (六 味 地 黄 丸)

liù wèi dì huáng wán

Radix rehmanniae, Cornus, Dioscoreae rhizoma, rhizoma alisma orientalis, Peony, Poria

Ma chi xian he ji (马 齿 苋 合 剂)

mǎ chǐ xiàn hé jì

Purslane, Isatidis folium, dandelion

Ma zi ren wan (麻 子 仁 丸)

má zǐ rén wán

Cannabis semen, Peony, Aurantii fructus immaturus, rhubarb, Magnoliae officinalis cortex, almonds

Mai wei di huang tang (麦 味 地 黄 汤)

mài wèi dì huáng tāng

Radix rehmanniae, Cornus, Moutan cortex, alisma, Poria cocos Wolf, Dioscoreae rhizoma, Schisandrae chinensis frucuts, Ophiopogonis radix

Niu bang jie ji tang (牛 蒡 解 肌 汤)

niú bàng jiě jī tāng

Arctium lappa, mint, Schizonepetae herba, Forsythia suspensa, gardenia, Moutan cortex, Dendrobium, ginseng, Prunella Vulgaris

Nuan gan jian (暖 肝 煎)

nuǎn gān jiān

Angelica sinensis, lycium barbarum, Poria, cumin, cinnamon, Aquilariae lignum resinatum

Pi yue ma ren wan (脾 约 麻 仁 丸)

pí yuē má rén wán

Cannabis semen, Peony, Aurantii fructus immaturus, rhubarb, Magnoliae officinalis cortex, almonds

Pi zhi gao (皮 脂 膏)

pí zhī gāo

Indigo naturalis, Phellodendri chinensis cortex, calcined gypsum, volatile oil obtained from the baked nitrate cowhide fume

Qi bao mei ran dan (七 宝 美 髯 丹)

qī bǎo měi rán dān

Fleece-flower root, Poria, Achyranthes, angelica, medlar, dodder, psoralen

Qi fu yin (七 福 饮)

qī fú yǐn

Ginseng, Angelicae sinensis radix, Atractylodis macrocephalae rhizoma, Rehmanniae radix praeparata, Glycyrrizae radix praeparata cum melle, jujube kernel, Aconiti lateralis radix praeparata

Qi san dan (七 三 丹)

qī sān dān

Plaster, hydrargrum oxydatum crudum

Qian lie xian tang (前 列 腺 汤)

qián liè xiàn tāng

Salviae miltiorrhizae radix, Zeeland, red peony, peach kernel, safflower, frankincense, myrrh, Vaccariae semen, Citri reticulatae pericarpium viride, Meliae fructus, cumin, Angelicae dahuricae radix, Patrinia herba, dandelion

Qin lian er mu wan (芩 连 二 母 丸)

qín lián èr mǔ wán

Coptidis rhizoma, Scutellariae radix, anemarrhena, Fritillaria, Chuanxiong rhizoma, Angelicae sinensis radix, white peony root, Rehmanniae radix, Rehmanniae radix praeparata, Typhae pollen, Saigae tataricae cornu, Lycii cortex, licorice

Qing dai gao (青 黛 膏)

Qīng dài gāo

Indigo naturalis, gypsum, talc, Phellodendri chinensis cortex, Vaseline

Qing fei yin (清 肺 饮)

qīng fèi yǐn

Poris cocos, Scutellariae radix, Mori cortex, Ophiopogonis radix, Gardeniae fructus, Akebia caulis

Qing gan lu hui wan (清 肝 芦 荟 丸)
qīng gān lú huì wán

Chuanxiong rhizoma, Radix angelicae sinensis, Radix paeoniae Alba, Rehmanniae radix, citri reticulatae pericarpium viride, Aloe Vera extract, kelp, Notarchus leachii cirrosus Stimpson, licorice, Gleditsiae abnormalis fructus, coptis chinensis

Qing gu san (清 骨 散)
qīng gǔ sàn

Bupleuri radix, Gentianae macrophyllae radix, turtle armor, Lycii cortex, Artemisiae annuae herba, Anemarrhenae rhizoma, licorice

Qing hao bie jia tang (青 蒿 鳖 甲 汤)
qīng hāo biē jiǎ tāng

Artemisiae annuae herba, Anemarrhenae rhizoma, Rehmanniae radix, turtle armor, Moutan cortex

Qing hao su (青 蒿 素)
qīng hāo sù

Artemisinin

Qing jin hua tan tang (清 金 化 痰 汤)
qīng jīn huà tán tāng

Radix scutellariae, gardenia, Plantycodonis radix, Ophiopogonis radix, Trichosanthis semen, Fritillariae cirrhosae bulbus, Ophiopogonis radix, Citri exocarpium rubrum, Poria, Mori cortex, Anemarrhenae rhizome, Radix glycyrrhiza uralensis

Run chang tang (润 肠 汤)
rùn cháng tāng

Cannabis semen, Sesami nigrum semen, Peach kernel, Herba schizonepetae spike

San ao tang (三 拗 汤)
sān ào tāng

Ephedra, almond, licorice

San miao wan (三 妙 丸)
sān miào wán

Atractylodes lancea, Phellodendron chinense, Achyranthes bidentata

Sang xing tang (桑 杏 汤)

sāng xìng tāng

Mulberry leaf, almond, Radix glehniae, Fritillaria, fragrant with black bean sauce, gardenia skin, pear skin

Sheng mai yin (生 脉 饮)

shēng mò yǐn

Ginseng, ophiopogon root, schisandra chinensis

Shi hui san (十 灰 散)

shí huī sàn

Cirsii japonica herba, Cirsii herba, Lotus leaf, platycladi cacumen, imperatae rhizoma, Rubiae radix et rhizoma, rhubarb, gardenia, Moutan cortex, Arecae pericarpium

Shi jun zi san (使 君 子 散)

shǐ jun1 zǐ sàn

Quisqualis, liquorice, Fructus ulmi macrocarpae preparatus, Meliae semen

Shi quan da bu tang (十 全 大 补 汤)

shí quán dà bǔ tāng

Ginseng, cinnamon, Chuanxiong rhizoma, Radix rehmanniae, Poria, white atractylodes Rhizome, licorice, Astragalus, Angelicae sinensis radix, White Peony, ginger, jujube

Shi quan liu qi yin (十 全 流 气 饮)

shí quán liú qì yǐn

Orange peel, red Poria, Radix linderae, Chuanxiong rhizoma, Radix angelicae sinensis, Radix paeoniae Alba, Cyperus, citri reticulatae pericarpium viride, Radix glycyrrhiza uralensis, Radix aucklandiae

Shi wei san (石 韦 散)

shí wéi sàn

Tetrapanacis medulia, Pyrrosiae folium, vaccaria, talc, Radix glycyrrhiza uralensis, Radix angelicae sinensis, rhizoma atractylodis macrocephalae, gypsophila, Paeonia lactiflora, Malvae fructus

Shuang bai san (双 柏 散)

shuāng bǎi sàn

Rhubarb, mint, Phellodendri chinensis cortex, eupatorium, platycladus orientalis

Si hai shu yu wan (四 海 舒 郁 丸)

sì   hǎi   shū   yù   wán

Aristolochia debilis Sieb, orange peel, sea clams powder, kelp, seaweed, Laminariae thallus, cuttlebone

Si huang gao (四 黄 膏)

sì   huáng   gāo

Coptis, rhubarb, Phellodendri chinensis cortex, skullcap

Si qi tang (四 七 汤)

sì   qī   tāng

Pinellia ternata, Poria, perilla leaves, Magnoliae officinalis cortex

Si wu tang (四 物 汤)

sì   wù   tāng

White Peony, Angelica sinensis, Radix rehmanniae, Chuanxiong rhizoma

Suan zao ren tang (酸 枣 仁 汤)

suān   zǎo   rén   tāng

Semen Ziziphi spinosae, Poria, Anemarrhena, Chuanxiong rhizoma, licorice

Tao hong si wu tang (桃 红 四 物 汤)

táo   hóng   sì   wù   tāng

Rehmanniae radix praeparata, Angelicae sinensis radix, root of herbaceous peony, rhizome of Ligusticum wallichii, peach kernel, safflower

Tiao ying yin (调 营 饮)

tiáo   yíng   yǐn

Radix paeoniae Rubra, Chuanxiong rhizoma, Radix angelicae sinensis, rhizoma curcumae, corydalis, betel nuts, corn cockle, tinglizi, Mori cortex, Radix salviae miltiorrhizae, Radix et rhizoma Rhei

Tiao yuan shen qi wan (调 元 肾 气 丸)

tiáo   yuán   shèn   qì   wán

Rehmannia, cornus, rhizoma dioscoreae, Peony, white Tuckahoe, ginseng, Radix angelicae sinensis, rhizoma alisma orientalis, Ophiopogonis radix, keel, cortex lycii, Radix aucklandiae, Amomum villosum, Phellodendri chinensis cortex, anemarrhena asphodeloides

Tong qi san jian wan (通 气 散 坚 丸)

tōng　qì　sàn　jiān　wán

Citri reticulatae pericarpium, pinellia, Poris cocos, licorice, Acori tatarinowii rhizoma, Aurantii fructus immaturus, ginseng, Arisaema cum bile, radix trichosanthes kirilowii, Platycodonis radix, rhizome Ligusticum wallichii, seaweed, Angelicae sinensis radix, fritillaria, Cyperi rhizoma, Scutellariae radix

Tu jin pi ding (土 槿 皮 酊)

tǔ　jǐn　pí　dǐng

Pseudolaricis cortex, Mylabris, alcohol

Wang shi lian po yin (王 氏 连 朴 饮)

wáng　shì　lián　pǔ　yǐn

Magnoliae officinalis cortex, Coptidis rhizoma, Acori tatarinowii rhizoma, Pinellia, Sojae semen praeparatum, Phragmitis rhizoma

Wen dan tang (温 胆 汤)

wēn　dǎn　tāng

Pinellia ternata, Bambusae caulis in taenias, Aurantii fructus immaturus, orange peel, licorice, Poria, ginger, jujube

Wu bei zi san (五 倍 子 散)

wǔ　bèi　zǐ　sàn

Gall nut, hops

Wu bei zi tang (五 倍 子 汤)

wǔ　bèi　zǐ　tāng

Gall nut, Mirabilitum, Taxilli herba, lotus room, nepeta japonica

Wu bi shan yao wan (无 比 山 药 丸)

Dogwood, alisma orientalis, Radix rehmanniae, Poria, Morinda, Achyranthes bidentata, Halloysitum rubrum, Yam, eucommia ulmoides, Dodder, Cistanche deserticola, schisandra chinensis

Wu miao shui xian gao (五 妙 水 仙 膏)

wǔ　miào　shuǐ　xiān　gāo

Phellodendri chinensis cortex, Arnebiae radix, gall nut

Wu shen tang (五 神 汤)

wǔ shén tāng

Poria cocos, plantain, Flos lonicerae, Radix achyranthis bidentatae, Viola yedoensis Makino

Wu wu dan (五 五 丹)

Plaster, Hydrargyrum oxydatum crudum

Xian tian da zao wan (先 天 大 造 丸)

xiān tiān dà zào wán

Placenta, Rehmannia, Angelicae sinensis radix, Poria, ginseng, Chinese wolfberry, dodder, Cistanche, Polygonati rhizoma, Atractylodis macrocephalae rhizoma, Polygonum multiflorum, Cyathulae radix, Curculigo, Drynaria, Morindae officinalis radix, Fructus psoraleae, Polygala, Aucklandiae radix, salt, cloves, black jujube meat

Xiang bei yang ying tang (香 贝 养 营 汤)

xiāng bèi yǎng yíng tāng

White atractylodes Rhizome, ginseng, Poria, Citri reticulatae pericarpium, Radix rehmanniae, Chuanxiong rhizoma, Radix angelicae sinensis, Fritillaria, Cyperus, White Peony root, platycodon grandiflorum, licorice, ginger, jujube

Xiao er hua shi tang (小 儿 化 湿 汤)

xiǎo ér huà shī tāng

Atractylodis rhizoma, Citri reticulatae pericarpium, Poris cocos, Alismatis rhizoma, Hordei fructus germinatus, liuyisan (talc and liquorice)

Xiao feng dao chi tang (消 风 导 赤 汤)

xiāo fēng dǎo chì tāng

Rehmanniae radix, red Poria, arctium lappa, cortex dictamni, honeysuckle, mint, akebia, rhizoma coptidis, Radix glycyrrhiza uralensis, Junci medulla

Xiao he wan (消 核 丸)

xiāo hé wán

Orange, red Poria, rhubarb, Hypericum perforatum, scutellaria, Gardeniae fructus, pinellia, oysters, Typhae pollen, platycodon grandiflorum, trichosanthes, Bombyx batryticatus

Xiao ji yin zi (小 蓟 饮 子)
xiǎo   jì   yǐn   zǐ
Dried rehmannia, Cirsii herba, talc, Akebiae caulis, Typhae pollen, lotus-root joints, Lophatheri herba, Angelicae sinensis radix, mountain gardenia, roasted licorice

Xiao jin dan (小 金 丹)
xiǎo   jīn   dān
Liquidambaris resina, Aconiti kusnezoffii radix, Momordicae semen, Pheretima, Trogopterus dung, myrrh, Angelicae sinensis radix, frankincense, musk, ink charcoal

Xiao li wan (消 疬 丸)
xiāo   lì   wán
Prunella, forsythia, castor kernel

Xiao yao lou bei san (逍 遥 蒌 贝 散)
xiāo   yáo   lóu   bèi   sàn
Bupleurum chinensis, Angelicae sinensis radix, root of herbaceous peony, Poris cocos, Atractylodis macrocephalae rhizoma, Chinese trichosanthes, fritillaria, pinellia, Arisaematis rhizoma, fresh oyster, mountain arrowhead

Xiao yao san (逍 遥 散)
xiāo   yáo   sàn
Licorice, Angelica sinensis, bupleurum, White Peony, atractylodes macrocephala, Poria cocos, mint

Xie re tang (泻 热 汤)
xiè   rè   tāng
Chinese goldthread rhizome, Scutellariae radix, weeping forsythia, Angelicae sinensis radix, Akebia caulis, licorice

Xie xin tang (泻 心 汤)
xiè   xīn   tāng
Rhubarb, coptis chinensis, Radix scutellariae

Xin yi qing fei yin (辛 夷 清 肺 饮)
xīn   yí   qīng   fèi   yǐn
Magnoliae officinalis cortex, scutellaria, Gardeniae fructus, Ophiopogonis radix, lilies, gypsum, anemarrhena, licorice, loquat leaf, Black Cohosh

Yang he jie ning gao (阳 和 解 凝 膏)
yáng   hé   jiě   níng   gāo

Fresh burdock grass, fresh herb of Tuberculate speranskia, Aconiti radix, Cinnamomi ramulus, rhubarb, Angelicae sinensis radix, cinnamon, Aconiti kusnezoffii radix, Aconiti lateralis radix, earthworm, Bombyx batryticatus, red peony, Angelicae dahuricae radix, Ampelopsis radix, Bletillae rhizome, Chuanxiong rhizome, Dipsacus, Saposhnikoviae radix, Trogopterus dung, Aucklandiae radix, citron, orange peel, Cinnamomi cortex, frankincense, myrrh, storax oil, musk

Yang he tang (阳 和 汤)
yáng   hé   tāng

Rehmanniae radix praeparata, Cinnamomi cortex, Ephedrae herba, Cervi cormus colla, sinapis alba, Zingiberis rhizoma praeparata, licorice

You gui yin (右 归 饮)
yòu   guī   yǐn

Rehmanniae radix praeparata, Chinese Yam, Cornus, Lucii fructus, Radix glycyrrhiza uralensis, eucommia ulmoides, cinnamon, aconite

Yu lu gao (玉 露 膏)
yù   lù   gāo

Lotus leaf, Vaseline

Zang lian wan (脏 连 丸)
zāng   lián   wán

Radix scutellariae, rhizoma coptidis, Radix rehmanniae, Radix paeoniae Rubra, Angelica sinensis, Sophorae fructus, Sophorae flos, Schizonepetae spica, Sanguisorbae radix carbonisata, donkey-hide gelatin

Zhi bao dan (至 宝 丹)
zhì   bǎo   dān

Bubali cornu, cinnabar, realgar, tortoiseshell crumbs, amber, musk, Borneol, gold foil, silver foil, bezoar, benzoin

Zhi chuang ding (痔 疮 锭)
zhì   chuāng   dìng

Belladonna fluid extract, Gallic acid bismuth, epinephrine

Zhi sou san (止 嗽 散)

zhǐ   sòu   sàn

Platycodon grandiflorum, Schizonepetae herba, Aster, Radix stemonae, Cynanchi stauntonii rhizoma et radix, liquorice, orange peel

Zhi tong ru shen tang (止 痛 如 神 汤)

zhǐ   tòng   rú   shén   tāng

Gentianae macrophyllae radix, peach kernel, Chinese honey locust, Atractylodis rhizoma, Saposhnikoviae radix, Phellodendri chinensis cortex, Angelicae sinensis radix, Alismatis rhizoma, betel nut, Chinese rhubarb

Zhong man fen xiao wan (中 满 分 消 丸)

zhōng   mǎn   fèn   xiāo   wán

Ginseng, rhizoma atractylodis macrocephalae, Poria, Glycyrrhizae radix praeparata cum melle, Polyporus umbellatus, pinellia, orange peel, ginger, turmeric, Amomum villosum, Alismati rhizoma, rhizoma anemarrhenae, Scutellariae radix, rhizoma coptidis, fructus aurantii immaturus, Magnoliae officinalis cortex

Zhu sha an shen wan (朱 砂 安 神 丸)

zhū   shā   ān   shén   wán

Cinnabar, coptis, rehmannia, Angelicae sinensis radix, licorice

Zhu ye huang qi tang (竹 叶 黄 芪 汤)

zhú   yè   huáng   qí   tāng

Ginseng, Astragalus, calcined gypsum, pinellia, ophiopogon root, White Peony root, Chuanxiong rhizoma, Radix angelicae sinensis, Radix scutellariae, Radix glycyrrhiza uralensis, Lophatheri herba, ginger, Junci medulla

Zi jin ding (紫 金 锭)

zǐ   jīn   ding

Knoxiae radix, Cremastrae pseudobulbus, leptochloa cream, Galla chinensis, musk, cinnabar, realgar

Zi xue dan (紫 雪 丹)

zǐ   xuě   dān

Gypsum fibrosum, Magnetitum, Gypsum rubrum, talc, powdered buffalo horn extract, Saigae tataricae cornu, Aquilariae lignum resinatum,

Aucklandiae radix, Scrophulariae radix, liquorice, cloves, Natrii sulfas, saltpetre, musk, cinnabar, Cimicifugae rhizoma

Zi yin chu shi tang (滋　阴　除　湿　汤)

zī　　yīn　　chú　　shī　　tāng

Rhizome of Ligusticum wallichii, Angelicae sinensis radix, root of herbaceous peony, Rehmanniae radix praeparata, bupleurum chinensis, Scutellariae radix, Citri reticulatae pericarpium, Anemarrhenae rhizoma, fritillaria, Alismatis rhizoma, Lycii cortex, licorice

BIBLIOGRAPHY

Antsaklis, P.J. and Michel, A. *Linear Systems*. McGraw-Hill Higher Education: New York, 1997.

Bauer, B. (ed.). *Mayo Clinic Book of Alternative Medicine*. Time Inc: New York, 2007.

Bensky, D., Clavey, S. and Stoger, E. *Chinese Herbal Medicine: Materia Medica. 3rd edition*. Eastland Press: Seattle, 2004.

Huang, K.C. *The Pharmacology of Chinese Herbs*. CRC Press: Boca Raton, 1999.

Ko, R.J. A U.S. perspective on the adverse reactions from Traditional Chinese Medicine. *J. Chin. Med. Assoc.* 67: 109–116, 2004.

Lin, J.G. (ed.). *Medical Terminology Dictionary of Western Medicine and Chinese Medicine*. People's Public Health Publishing House: Beijing, 2002.

Liu, C. and Tseng, A. *Chinese Herbal Medicine: Modern Applications of Traditional Formulas*. CRC Press: Boca Raton, 2005.

Luenberger, D.C. *Introduction to Dynamic Systems*. John Wiley & Sons Inc: New York, 1979.

Need, G. *Blood Stasis: China's Classical Concept in Modern Medicine*. Elsevier: New York, 2007.

Peilin, S. (ed.). *The Treatment of Pain with Chinese Herbs and Acupuncture*. Churchill Livingston: New York, 2002.

Rossi, E. *Shen: Psycho-Emotional Aspects of Chinese Medicine*. Elsevier: New York, 2007.

Sastry, S. *Nonlinear Systems: Analysis, Stability, and Control*. Springer-Verlag: New York, 1999.

Scheid, V. *Currents of Tradition in Chinese Medicine: 1626–2006*. Eastland Press: Seattle, 2007.

Textbook Committee. *Textbook of Chinese Medicine*. Shanghai Science and Technology Publishing House: Shanghai, 1984.

Textbook Committee. *Planned Textbook of Chinese Medicine*. Shanghai Science and Technology Publishing House: Shanghai, 1994.

Xu, B. Recommendation on Chinese Medicine in the United States. To White House Commission on Complementary and Alternative Medicine Policy. ACMA Publication, Dec 1, 2001. http://www.AmericanChineseMedicineAssociation.org.

Xu, B. Fundamental characteristics of Chinese Medicine: Holism and Treatments Based on CM Diagnosis. ACMA Publication, Feb 1, 2003. http://www.AmericanChineseMedicineAssociation.org.

Xu, B. Mathematical herbal medicine. *Acupuncture Today,* 6: 2005.

Yuan, C.S., Bieber, E.J. and Bauer, B.A. (eds.). *Textbook of Complementary and Alternative Medicine, 2nd Edition*. Informa Healthcare: New York, 2006.

Index